Nordic Walking

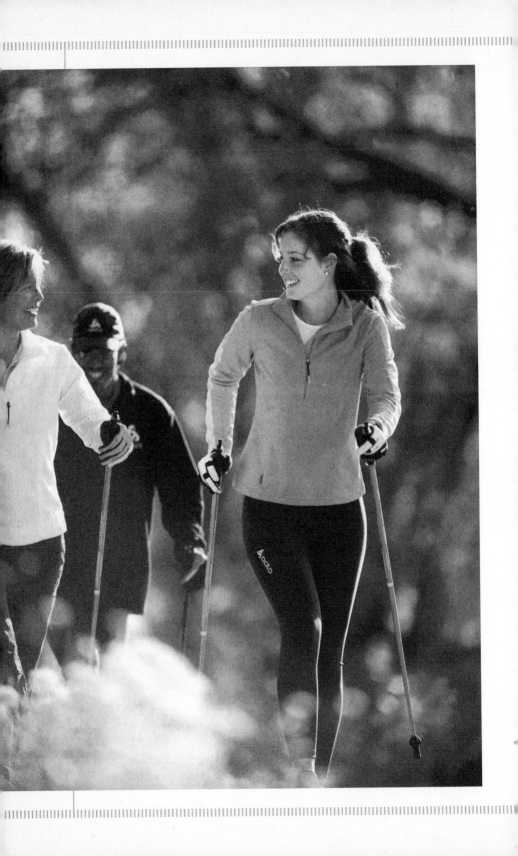

Nordic Walking

The Complete Guide to Health, Fitness and Fun

Claire Walter

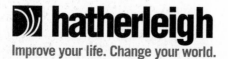

Improve your life. Change your world.

Hatherleigh Press
5-22 46ᵗʰ Avenue, Suite 200
Long Island City, NY 11101
www.hatherleighpress.com

Library of Congress Cataloging-in-Publication Data

Walter, Claire.
Nordic walking : the new way to health, fitness and fun / Claire Walter.
p. cm.
ISBN 978-1-57826-269-4 (pbk. : alk. paper) 1. Fitness walking. I. Title.
GV502.W35 2008
613.7'176--dc22
2008052483

Nordic Walking is available for bulk purchase, special promotions, and premiums. For information on reselling and special purchase opportunities, call 1-800-528-2550 and ask for the Special Sales Manager.

Interior design by Nick Macagnone
Cover design by Christopher Tobias
Photography by Catarina Astrom

Images on pages 116, 130, 147 courtesy of www.anwa.us/ ANWA—the American Nordic Walking Association
Images on pages ii, xxii, 129, 140 courtesy of Exel
Images on pages 19, 37, and 70 courtesy of Exerstrider®
Images on pages 30 courtesy of Fittrek
Image on page 149 courtesy of FlashPRO
Image on page 10 courtesy of FootePath
Image on page 118 courtesy of Gymstick
Images on pages 41, 56, 80 courtesy of Keenfit
Image on page 158 courtesy of Komperdell
Images on pages 35, 46 courtesy of Claire Walter

10 9 8 7 6 5 4 3 2 1
Printed in United States

Disclaimer

This book is for informational purposes only for the new Nordic Walker or individual contemplating commencing Nordic Walking. As with other printed media containing equipment and instructional information on a fitness program or active sport, readers are advised to consult a physician or other medical professional before beginning to Nordic Walk. This is particularly true for people new to exercise and fitness activities, or those who have chronic or temporary medical conditions that might be helped by Nordic Walking. There are no warranties, either express or implied, that the material in this book is anything other than informational. Readers who sign up for a Nordic Walking program, purchase or rent poles, join a group or organization, or in any way use the information in this book do so at their own risk. Neither Hatherleigh Press nor the author assumes any liability for illness or injury that may arise from the use of this book. Use or information contained in this book carries the user's assumption of risk. The reader and Nordic Walking practitioner is solely responsible for his or her Nordic Walking actions.

Acknowledgments

Nordic Walking is such a new activity in North America that I feel like thanking everyone who participates—instructors, guides, long-time enthusiasts and just regular people who have recently picked up poles and started walking to satisfy whatever their personal goals might be. I have met a few in person, interviewed others by phone, corresponded with many more by e-mail and/or learned of the interests and concerns of still others via comments to my posts on my Nordic Walking blog (http://nordic-walking-usa.blogspot.com). A list of all the individuals who helped me sort out the puzzle pieces that a growing activity like Nordic Walking presents would comprise another chapter, which is the last thing the patient folks at Hatherleigh Press— June Eding, Editor; Anna Krusinski, Associate Editor—would want to see from me.

Dedication

To my husband, Ral Sandberg, who—inspired by Dave Barry who described power walking as "dork walking"—initially made merry and called Nordic Walking, "dork walking with sticks," but has since come around and acknowledged its benefits and its pleasure.

Contents

Preface

I first encountered Nordic Walking in September 2005 in the Alpine resort of Mürren, Switzerland. I was there for some hiking with travel writer colleagues following a convention in St. Moritz. When I saw Nordic Walking on the hotel's program of available activities and asked what it was, I was told "walking with poles," in hindsight an accurate but woefully incomplete description—and certainly not enough motivation to trade in my trekking poles for Nordic Walking poles and learn more.

Several friends and I trekked for overnight stays in remote hotels quite apart from Mürren, so we never encountered the Nordic Walkers. When we returned from our trek a few days later, the Nordic Walking group at our hotel bubbled over with chatty enthusiasm. Over drinks and at the dinner table, they enthused relentlessly. Nordic Walking was fun. Nordic Walking was a fantastic workout. Nordic Walking made them feel good. Nordic Walking was energizing. Nordic Walking was great. I ought to try it right away, they suggested, because they knew that I would love it too. I couldn't, because I had a train to catch, but every European whom I talked to about it during the next week seemed astonished that I hadn't known about this fitness phenomenon.

The following summer, I finally had the opportunity to pick up a pair of Nordic Walking poles at Devil's Thumb Ranch in Colorado, one of the first resorts in the country to recognize its potential. I'm not naturally athletic, but as a long-time Alpine and cross-country skier, snowshoer and hiker who has used trekking poles for a number of years, I am accustomed to poles. Still, Nordic Walking didn't come to me instantly. In hindsight, when I first used special Nordic Walking poles, I was planting them more like trekking poles. The woman who led DTR's initial Nordic Walks was then fairly recently trained herself and had more than just me to pay attention to. Still, after an hour and a half of not doing it quite right, I was overcome with a powerful sense that Nordic Walking is something special. I started reading about it, researched it some more, wrote about it a bit and joined local introductory classes whenever I could. I played around with my poles, and my so-called technique kept feeling marginally better, but not quite right. As I wrote earlier, I'm neither a natural athlete—nor am I a quick study.

It all clicked for me in spring of 2007, when Gottfried Kürmer came to town. In addition to his considerable credentials as an athlete and a trainer in his native Austria, he had been certified as an International Nordic Walking Association's Master Coach, the highest certification level. Bernd Zimmerman, founder of the American Nordic Walking Association (ANWA), and Gottfried invited me to join ANWA's Basic Instructor certification class, an eight-hour workshop that prepares people to teach Nordic Walking at an introductory level. My classmates included a personal trainer, an office manager who had already lost more than 100 pounds and wanted to encourage others to do the same with exercise as well as dieting, a certified nurse-practitioner specializing in helping older adults to become and stay active, and a 74-year-old low-income senior whose tuition was subsidized by a social-services agency so that she could help other local seniors enjoy the benefits of Nordic Walking. I took the course as a big part of the research for this book. Learning to teach catapulted me past a technique problem where I had been stuck. Previously, my foot and arm movements and the position of the pole plant were all right—or at least I believed they were. But the timing or rhythm of the pole plant coupled with opening the hand, reaching the arm back far enough and catching the pole grip again as the arm moved forward was off. I knew I was doing something wrong, but I couldn't self-correct.

About halfway through the day, I got it, and as soon as I did, I took off as if my afterburners fired up. My pace picked up, and the entire Nordic Walking motion sequence suddenly felt right. My movements felt fluid and free, powerful and invigorating. Gottfried didn't point out any mistakes, so I'm guessing my progress was palpable. His workshop helped me past the plateau on which I, as a new and still sometime Nordic Walker, had been stuck. And, as bonus, I am now the proud holder of ANWA certification as a Nordic Walking instructor. Will I ever teach? Not likely, but in learning to teach, my skill level skyrocketed. In the months and miles that followed, I am certain that my technique has eroded from the ANWA ideal, but I don't really think it matters, because I use my poles energetically and maximize my daily walk.

In the process of all this, the idea for this book unfolded. Very little has been written about Nordic Walking, and the very few available books on the subject have been done by Nordic Walking instructors and trainers—people with a high level of knowledge and personal fitness and experience in teaching the fine points of Nordic Walking. However, each author seems to have a bit of an agenda to promote these fine points as established by a particular association or a particular pole manufacturer. Is one really "better" than the others, or are they merely different? I am no position to judge the way a physiologist might, but I contend that the most important thing is for people to start doing it with as much professional instruction and guidance as possible, and then keep on doing it until it is an ingrained fitness habit. Even though I am now certified, I am not a fitness professional—and I don't even play one on television. I am a writer and now a Nordic Walking enthusiast. When I began to write this book, my goals were to tell new Nordic Walkers all the small details that I had been curious about and also to share information that I turned up during my research. I hope I have done so. I present you with what I have gleaned and leave it to you to make your Nordic Walking choices. I also maintain a blog at http://nordic-walking-usa.blogspot.com. I invite you to visit often, because I plan to continue following developments in the Nordic Walking world.

Claire Walter
Boulder, Colorado
March 2009

Introduction

Finland has given us Marimekko fabrics, Iittala porcelain, Nokia cell phones and sauvakävely. *Sauvakävely?* Literally translated as pole walking, it is, at its most basic, fitness-walking using a pair of lightweight poles. Out of a population of roughly 5,225,000, half a million Finns participate in "pole walking." If Americans did so at the same level, roughly 27 million people would be striding across the countryside with poles.

The first European steps of what would some years later be called Nordic Walking were taken by members of Finnish cross-country ski racers as part of centennial celebrations honoring the birth of Professor Lauri "Tahko" Pikhala, a national sports pioneer. During a particularly snowless January in Helsinki, conditions mandated scrapping the original idea of skiing to the event, so cross-country skiers grabbed their Nordic poles and strode down the route of the procession. A local newspaper called *Helsingen Sanomat* reported, "The Nordic Walking pioneers recognized pretty soon that they had invented an exercise discipline that was eminently well suited to the autumn and to the snow-starved winters of Southern Finland."

Rooted in summer dryland training used in the 1930s by Finnish cross-country skiers and brought to attention by the Pikhala celebration, it morphed into a general fitness activity. Its popularity skyrocketed following the introduction of specially designed poles and of specific technique. Fitness-walking and training with poles was codified and developed by Marko Kantaneva. He first called it sauvakävely, which translates as "pole walking" and later came up with the more international name, Nordic Walking. He also defined various terms involved in the activity, all at the behest of Finnish ski-pole manufacturer Exel Oy. Exel introduced activity-specific poles for this new activity that Kantaneva codified, and began giving a major marketing push to its poles and the technique in 1997. Soon leading ski-pole makers in other European countries, such as LEKI in Germany and Swix in Norway, began making special Nordic Walking poles too. Within a few years, sporting goods stores were stocking them, people were buying them and instructors were popping up in major cities and resort villages alike to teach Nordic Walking. It rapidly spread to the Scandinavian countries of Norway, Sweden and Denmark, and down into Germany, Austria and Switzerland, where it became quite the fitness rage. In Great Britain, which is laced with public footpaths, Nordic Walking has gained many adherents. Nordic Walking enthusiasts can also be found now in Japan, France, Italy, the Benelux countries and Iceland. In Europe, Nordic Walking is usually considered to be a sport—much like recreational (and often high-level) running, cycling, swimming and skiing—and also a contributor to overall wellness. In fact, national health plans in European countries often cover Nordic Walking instruction and poles as part of preventive medicine. No one has kept track of exactly how many people Nordic Walk at least once a week, but participation is estimated to be about 6 million in Europe at this writing in 2008. By 2010, the number of Nordic Walkers could soar to 10 million.

Fitness-walking with poles developed in something of parallel universes on either side of the Atlantic. While European Nordic Walking came from the cross-country ski tradition, many pioneers in the United States and Canada had been either serious runners or fitness professionals. Trainers and other pros liked the combination of aerobic and muscle benefits gained by energetic walking with poles. Runners found this low-impact activity to be less stressful on their aching joints than running. Once they began training with poles, they noticed that it carried other benefits as well. Some of these runners-turned-pioneering-pole-walkers developed their own techniques and equipment, and began to spread the gospel but without the marketing might of brand-name European companies that promoted growth there.

The American development of fitness-walking with poles was more intentional than accidental. In 1986, a competitive runner from Wisconsin named Tom Rutlin developed a heel spur and started using his cross-country ski poles to enable him to maintain his aerobic conditioning. He understood and liked everything about fitness-walking with poles that we now take as common knowledge: total body workout to develop a higher level of cardiovascular health, endurance, joint flexibility, etc. Even after he recovered from the heel spur, he never returned to running, but continued to refine his new walking epiphany. In 1988, he introduced Exerstrider poles and a fitness-walking technique that he called Exerstriding. His pioneering innovations were deliberate and carefully thought-out efforts to address specific problems like those he himself had faced. He introduced Exerstrider strapless poles and launched a company.

The original Exerstrider pole, a one-piece model, is still available, and adjustable poles are now also offered. Exerstriders remain nearly unique in a product category in which other poles feature straps of various types—an exception being Fittrek (see page 48) which offers one model with a strapless option. Rutlin designed his ERGO/SC grips for maximum comfort and what he describes as a "15-degree rear-flared design [that] allows a relaxed hand to control the grip while maintaining a comfortable, neutral wrist." Exerstrider's legions of fans like the fact that there is no chafing, which some users experience in hot weather when walking for a long time with poles that have straps. Another benefit cited by cold-weather walkers is that they can wear heavy gloves or even mittens without interference when the temperature plunges.

Interestingly, given the higher-profile European side of the sport's family, *Esquire* magazine's German edition was the first among major media to recognize Exerstriding. The February 1989 edition contained a short item specifically on Exerstriding. It called Rutlin's approach "Mit Schuhen und Stöcken" (with shoes and sticks) and tagged it as "der neue Trend aus USA" (which needs no translation). For more than two decades, Tom Rutlin has been passionate about growing the sport and fitness activity of walking with poles.

In North America, where it is still in its numerical infancy in terms of participation, we call it Nordic Walking, "Exerstriding" (after the very first pole company), SkiWalking (after another company founded later by Pete Edwards), pole walking, urban poling, balance walking (used by Foot Solutions stores) or other variations of these and similar names. While large companies with long sporting-equipment traditions put their design, manufacturing and marketing muscle behind it in Europe, individual entrepreneurs like Rutlin, Edwards, Dan Barrett of Fittrek and Jeff Lunde of Boomyah who followed have started businesses in North America and promoted fitness-walking with poles.

"What's in a name?" William Shakespeare asked. "That which we call a rose," he wrote in answer, "by any other name would smell as sweet." The many threads in the tapestry of fitness-walking with poles presented me with something of a dilemma, but I did have to settle on one set of terms for this book and eventually chose to use Nordic Walking and Nordic Walker. My use of Nordic Walking and Nordic Walker (capitalized) is not to be mistaken for an endorsement of any specific technique or product over another. Whatever it is called, fitness-walking with poles provides efficient aerobic exercise without gym membership, Lycra workout clothes, or pounding music. It offers an opportunity to get out of the house or office and exercise outdoors—and that's how American fitness enthusiasts tend to view it: as a fitness activity, one that has no place to grow but up.

Americans who love the promise of weight-loss magic respond to Nordic Walking statistics. Just as an example, walking with poles burns between about 20 and 45 percent more calories and increases oxygen consumption by up to 25 percent compared with walking at the same speed, on the same grade and over the same distance without poles. And if that wasn't enough, Nordic Walking is inexpensive and easy to learn. A set of poles and good walking shoes (which may be specifically made for Nordic Walking) are the only investments, and a little bit of coaching to help you imprint the correct movements is all there is to it. Many people enjoy the social aspect of participating in an organized Nordic Walking group or just going out with a spouse, partner or a friend or two. It's amazing how quickly the miles fly by, weight flies off and general health increases for people who become dedicated Nordic Walkers.

Nordic Walking crosses the boundaries of age and agility as well. Children love the fun of it (skipping with poles particularly appeals to them). Seniors can do it safely and comfortably. Runners and other well-conditioned athletes ratchet up their pace as part of a serious training regimen that is kind to the joints, and of course, those with competitive fever coursing through their veins enjoy racing with poles as well. And people rehabbing from sports and other injuries find Nordic Walking the best medicine to get back in shape without jeopardizing recuperation—in fact, it often aids healing. Again think about Europe, where Nordic Walking is considered a legitimate therapeutic treatment, and some government and private health plans cover courses and poles. For instance, Germany refunds hospital outpatients for their cost of attending certified Nordic Walking courses, and at least two Swiss health insurance plans include financial incentives paid to policyholders for NordicWalking courses. It has also been identified as the perfect fitness activity for aging baby boomers who want to stay famously fit or finally become so. Some want to relieve knees or backs that ache from years of running, mogul skiing, step aerobics or other impactful activities. Some will have had an injury or surgery, and are eager to get back to doing something active as soon as possible without making their situation worse. Some look in the mirror or squint at the bathroom scale and don't like what they see. Others have a medical scare and are told to shape up or else. It will be increasingly easy to do so, thanks to the growing corps of fitness instructors, personal trainers and even physical therapists trained as Nordic Walking instructors.

It was in the mid-1980s that Finnish pole manufacturer Exel hired Marko Kantaneva to design poles specifically for Nordic Walking. He did that and more, also laying the groundwork for the Finland-based International Nordic Walking Association, which Exel promoted. Especially in Europe, Kantaneva is generally credited with codifying technique, creating an instructional curriculum to teach it and setting standards for instructor certification at various levels. Soon, other European pole makers followed, perhaps tweaking the Exel progression and technique. Across the Atlantic, the aforementioned pioneering North Americans were developing some form of fitness-walking with poles, often with their own variations on technique as well as pole design.

In a sense, the confluence between the European- and American-born versions came when Europeans active in North America's sports and fitness communities began attempting to codify training and technique on this continent in the European mode. In 2005, Austrian-born Bernd Zimmermann established the American Nordic Walking Association as a national instructor training and certification organization and also to promote Nordic Walking. LEKI is an ANWA sponsor, but the organization is officially independent of all brands. Gerry Faderbauer, also originally from Austria, founded the Canadian Nordic Walking Association in 2006. CNWA markets its own brand of poles called Iwalk2. Like ANWA, CNWA trains and certifies instructors.

In some respects, Nordic Walking has developed along much the same pattern as the fitness industry, with more than one instructor training and certifying body, but pole manufacturers also continue to train instructors and devise their own variations on technique. LEKI and Exel remain European powerhouses, and smaller, entrepreneurial companies from both sides of the Atlantic have also developed their own technique specifics along with their pole designs. A number of the pole makers, big and small, run introductory workshops and often train their own instructors as well. The difference between "certified" and "trained" is a subtle one, and there are competent instructors with either credential. Some instructors, in fact, make the effort to be trained by a particular manufacturer and also to become certified by a national organization.

Now, sign up for a class, pick up a pair of poles and start Nordic

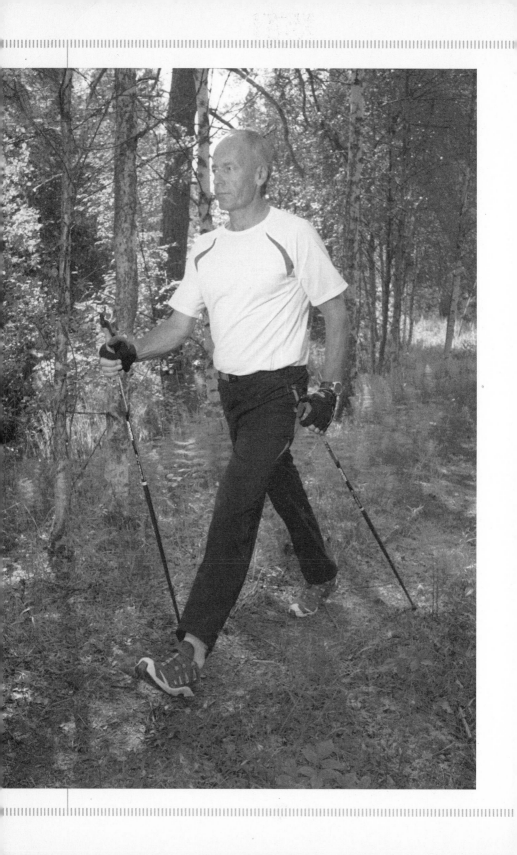

Nordic Walking
for Wellness

"Wellness" has entered our vocabulary as a word that emphasizes the positive aspects of health and fitness. Nordic Walking, a deceptively simple yet very effective form of fitness-walking with poles, offers everything that makes for an effective part of a wellness program. The learning curve for this complete workout is short, and it can be done virtually anywhere—on urban recreation paths, on suburban sidewalks or country lanes, on walking paths through the woods, on hiking trails or along sandy beaches. Necessary equipment is nothing more than special poles and proper shoes. From the first time you slip your hands through the pole straps, start out and get the hang of Nordic Walking's rhythm, you'll find it to be exhilarating, energizing and just plain fun. And because it's pleasurable as well as effective, it's easy to stick with.

More important, Nordic Walking is astonishingly beneficial for people at any level of fitness, even those with conditions that would seem to preclude many other forms of exercise. With just a little guidance, couch potatoes who are just getting started on a fitness routine can find it easy to learn proper and effective technique. Because Nordic Walking works both the upper and lower body, it strengthens the core —and that in turn contributes immeasurably to feelings of well-being, of good health, strength and suppleness. Walking enthusiasts find that it ratchets up their walks, burns significantly more calories than walking without poles, gets the heart pumping, and the lungs working. Runners whose knees have taken too many years of too much pounding find that this low-impact, high-results activity can prolong their running lives by giving them an aerobically challenging and less painful alternative activity. People recovering from a knee, ankle or hip injury or surgery find Nordic Walking an effective part of a rehabilitation program, because so much of the pressure is borne by the upper body, and some enlightened physical therapists are beginning to incorporate poles into rehabilitation programs. And seniors, even people of very advanced age, find Nordic Walking poles to be godsend because they provide stability, enabling them to stay physically active longer. There is also growing evidence that dedication to a demanding physical activity can help people overcome substance abuse or addiction problems.

The key to Nordic Walking has been the development of lightweight poles that loosely resemble cross-country ski poles, but with rubber tips for traction on pavement and pointed metal tips for dirt or gravel surfaces. Most models are designed so that the rubber tip is slipped over the metal one, but a few kinds of poles are designed with two-in-one flip tips that convert easily for use from one surface to another. Poles and other gear will be discussed in Chapters 2 and 3.

Start Moving For Good Health

Books, magazines, television and the Internet are full of advice on how to lose weight, how to lift your spirits, how to keep your bones healthy in order to stave off osteoporosis, how to lessen your chances of developing a host of diseases, how to retain your mobility and flexibility as you age and much more. Just think of how many how-to books and articles have you read that start with the importance of "regular exercise"—or often, "regular moderate exercise."

Study after study—as well as plain common sense—peg walking as extremely beneficial in addressing all of these health issues. Just plain walking, without poles, is considered a form of "moderate" exercise. According to a study cited in the American Medical Association's *Archives of Internal Medicine*, walking just 30 minutes a day most days of the week lengthens a person's life by an average of 1.3 years and increases the time without cardiovascular disease by an average 1.1 years compared to an inactive or low-activity lifestyle. Ratcheting up that moderate activity level to high, say with energetic Nordic Walking for longer periods, adds an average of 3.7 years of life and 3.3 years without cardiovascular disease.

While women have been the most enthusiastic converts to fitness-walking with poles, middle-age men are potentially the greatest beneficiaries. A seven-year study of 15,660 men (57 percent Caucasian and 43 percent African-American, with an average age of 59) found that those in the "very highly fit" category had a 70 percent lower death risk than those in the "low fit" category. Those considered moderately fit had about a 50 percent lower death risk compared with the low-fit group, according to Dr. Peter Kokkinos, director of an exercise testing lab at the Veterans Affairs Medical Center in Washington, DC, and lead author of the study published in early 2008 by *Circulation: Journal of the American Heart Association*. At the end of 7 years, 44 percent of the least-fit group died, 30 percent of the moderately fit, 15 percent of the highly fit and only 8 percent of the very highly fit.

Dr. Kokkinos suggested that "moderate fitness" isn't that difficult to achieve, saying, "You need to take a brisk walk for 30 minutes four to six times a week. It's not as easy as taking a pill, but let's be reasonable here." He added the increasing that activity into a fitter zone, which ultimately yields more benefits, doesn't take much more. He suggested jogging during part of that brisk walk. I'm no medical researcher—and I don't even play one on television—but adding poles and going for a brisk Nordic Walk for 30 minutes four to six times a week offers the same additional benefits without the stress to knees and ankles that even jogging might produce. Remember that the fitter you are, the longer you are likely to live—and your quality of life will be enhanced as well. So pick up those poles and get moving.

Now the disclaimer that you have seen on every recorded exercise program, whether on television, on tape or on CD and elsewhere: Check with your doctor before starting this or any exercise. Your doctor will probably cheer you on and encourage you to embark on regular Nordic Walking outings.

Getting to the Heart of the Matter

Anyone who has paid attention to the steady stream of television news reports, interviews with doctors on talk shows and commercials for medications has heard that heart attack and stroke, the two "silent killers," are the leading causes of death among Americans. Need more specific convincing? Noting that the number of Americans with type 2 diabetes (and related heart disease) has skyrocketed in the last half-century, a 2007 article in the American Heart Association's *Circulation* reported that so, too, has heart disease with attendant risk of heart attacks and strokes linked to the blood sugar illness. "The proportion of heart disease due to diabetes has increased about 60 percent over time," according to the lead author, Dr. Caroline S. Fox, a medical officer at the National Heart, Lung, and Blood Institute's Framingham Heart Study. "Compared with other risk factors for heart disease, diabetes is becoming more of an issue," she said. A predisposition to diabetes is bad. Being overweight worsens the risks.

Remember that diabetics either do not produce enough insulin or the cells ignore the insulin that is produced. Insulin is what converts sugar into energy, and in diabetics, if left untreated, sugar levels can soar, which is downright scary when you consider that common complications from diabetes are heart disease, blindness, nerve and kidney damage. In fact, 65 percent of all diabetics eventually die from heart disease or stroke, according to the American Heart Association.

Whether or not a person is diabetic, or even pre-diabetic, doctors and researchers now know that belly fat is also an indicator or precursor of heart attack and stroke. The good news is that with a half-hour of exercise per day and the loss of 10 to 15 pounds, you can reduce the risk of developing diabetes by over 58 percent and hopefully, a lot of that weight will come right off the gut. Diet, of course, impacts health in general and heart health in particular, but food choices and nutrition are beyond the scope of this book. Exercise-linked weight management is discussed below.

The American Heart Association, along with its sister organization, the American Stroke Association, is so concerned about the frightening increase in heart-related disease that it spearheads a motivational program called Start! The program calls on all Americans to change their lifestyles in order enjoy longer, more heart-healthy lives through walking and other positive habits. Recognizing how challenging it is for people to commit to and, more importantly stick to, the kind of physical activity necessary to control weight and lead that heart-healthy lifestyle, Start! keys in on walking, calling it "the easiest, most convenient form of activity — and it's free. You don't need special skills, the training of a marathon runner, or a membership at an expensive gym to benefit from walking." Everything that is true regarding the benefits of walking is compounded simply by adding specially designed poles, learning proper technique and becoming a Nordic Walker.

Benefits of Walking

The American Heart Association, which has not yet released a Nordic Walking-specific list at this writing, counsels the following benefits derived from walking in general for as little as 30 minutes a day:

For the body, walking helps to:
- Reduce the risk of heart disease by improving blood circulation throughout the body
- Keep weight under control
- Improve blood cholesterol levels
- Prevent and manage high blood pressure
- Prevent bone loss
- Boost energy levels
- Increase muscle strength, increasing the ability to do other physical activities

For the mind, walking helps to:
- Manage stress
- Release tension
- Improve the ability to fall asleep quickly and sleep well
- Improve self-image
- Counter anxiety and depression and increase enthusiasm and optimism

Weight Management

Weight management—whether as an end unto itself simply to look better or for preventive or other health reasons—is where Nordic Walking really shines. Americans are constantly assaulted by drug and supplement claims that promise rapid weight loss and diets that focus on or eliminate specific food categories (all protein, no carb, low carb, no fat, high fiber, etc.). However, nothing is a substitute for controlling caloric intake and engaging in regular exercise to reap lasting benefits. In short, controlling weight—whether as an effort to shed pounds or to maintain a healthy weight—requires a combination of diet and exercise. While Americans in general are fatter and "un-fitter" than ever, people are still susceptible to searching for the holy grail of quick and easy solutions to our overweight woes.

We read and see claims for radical diets and miracle drugs that make all sorts of too-good-to-be-true promises. Television commercials and print advertisements aside, look at the covers of leading magazines that run headlines like: "7 Ways to Lose 7 Pounds in 7 Days", "Take Off Ten by Thanksgiving", and "Hollywood Weight Loss Secrets." For most people, the result is a frustrating pounds-off/pounds-on loop. Many perpetual dieters have dual wardrobes of "fat clothes" and "thin clothes" that reflect this yo-yo routine of putting pounds on, taking pounds off, putting pounds on, taking pounds off.

To succeed, no matter what combination of diet and exercise is effective for you in losing weight and never finding it again, your body needs to utilize more calories than it takes in. Even people who obsessively count calories often don't know what they are counting. At its most fundamental level, a calorie is a scientific word for a unit of heat measure. It takes one calorie to raise one kilogram of water by one degree Celsius. For practical purposes, that translates in the human body to the way in which it converts what you have eaten into energy, both for its needs simply to maintain itself and also to fuel any activities that you do. When you take in more calories than your body consumes, you pack on pounds. When you burn more calories than you are taking in, your body turns to its fat stores for energy, and you begin to lose weight.

All food contains calories. The rule of thumb is 8 calories per gram of fat and 4 calories per gram of carbohydrate or protein. Figuring that a pound of body fat represents approximately 3,500 calories, most people can lose a pound a week just by lowering their caloric intake by 500 calories per day. Exercising burns additional calories. Individuals burn different amounts of calories, depending on their body weight, intensity and duration of their exercise, and other factors, so take all calorie-use charts as guidelines, not gospel. As a ballpark, however, if you watch your food intake and exercise moderately to burn just 500 calories a day, you can expect to shed about one pound per week. The average adult walking without poles burns about 280 calories per hour. Add poles, and that calorie burn increases to as much as 450 calories per hour. Nordic Walking at a moderate pace for as little as 3 hours a week burns 1,500 to 2,000 calories and provides a steady way to lose weight, even without dieting. If weight maintenance is your goal, Nordic Walking enables you to treat yourself to something sinfully delicious now and again without packing on additional pounds.

The Cooper Institute Study

"The Cooper Institute is dedicated to advancing the understanding of the relationship between living habits and health and to providing leadership in implementing these concepts to enhance the physical and emotional well-being of individuals."

In 2000, the highly regarded Cooper Institute of Dallas, Texas, conducted a study that Nordic Walking proponents love to quote and quote again and quote yet again. Tests done in the laboratory and in the field mimicked recreational walking. Test subjects covered the same distance at the same speed with and without poles indicated that Nordic Walking burns more calories and increases oxygen consumption by about 20 percent, increases the heart rate by 10 beats per minute and burns up to 46 percent more calories as compared to normal walking. The reason is that during normal walking without poles, about 70 percent of the body's muscle mass is engaged at any time. By contrast, because of the poling action, Nordic Walking engages 90 percent of the body's muscle mass. At the same time, the Cooper Institute study found, the rate of perceived exertion (RPE) is the same whether walking with or without poles. That means that Nordic Walkers don't feel as if they are working harder than people walking without poles. Since the benefit from Nordic Walking is greater that walking without poles, it provides, to quote the saying, more bang for your buck.

Overweight and Injured: The Connection

In a study of 42,304 adults who had suffered serious injuries between 1999 and 2002, researchers concluded that overweight individuals are more likely to be injured than those within a healthy weight range—and for the extremely obese, the risk was twice as high as for normal-weight individuals. RTI International, a leading international research firm in North Carolina, found a direct statistical correlation between body mass index (BMI) and injuries requiring medical attention. Overweight adults (BMI between 26 and 29) had a 15 percent greater risk of injury than normal-weight adults, and morbidly obese individuals (BMI of 40 or higher) had a whopping 48 percent greater risk.

These findings underscore studies of work-related injuries at Duke University that found the heaviest employees had filed workers' compensation claims at twice the rate of their fit co-workers. Duke researchers, studying nearly 12,000 university employees and people in its health system, additionally found that the fattest workers had 13 times more lost workdays because of work-related injuries than their fitter colleagues. Furthermore, their medical claims for injuries (most often to the back, wrist, arm, neck, shoulder, hip, knee and foot) were 7 times higher than their fit co-workers. Again, those with BMIs of 40 or greater had the highest rates of claims and the most lost workdays. Adding the greater probability of injury to the greater likelihood of disease provides yet another reason to pare down the pounds and shape up.

Nordic Walking would seem to be an ideal feature of any company-sponsored wellness program. Even those enlightened employers who are able to promote wellness must be mindful of possible accusations of discrimination based on weight or body type if such programs target the heaviest employees who are at the greatest risk of illness or injury. It's a catch-22. Companies should be most concerned for the health and productivity of their most overweight employees, yet those employees could file complaints of discrimination, which in turn would prevent the kind of program that could help them.

Exercise is the Secret of Wellness

Thinking about sickness and illness focuses on preventing the negative. Maintaining wellness and well-being focuses on the positive. Exercise can do both, and it's useful to understand the role that Nordic Walking can play in the general exercise and fitness scene. Here are some general comments that will help clarify general categories of exercise.

Aerobic exercise includes various types of physical activity that raise the heart rate in order to increase the blood supply and deliver oxygen to the muscles over an extended period. A stronger heart and stronger lungs mean that these vital organs are also healthier, which means that you are healthier overall. Examples of aerobic activities include brisk walking with or without poles, jogging, swimming, jumping rope, in-line skating with or without poles and cross-country skiing. In the gym, you might hear aerobic exercises referred to as cardio workouts. The bottom line, however, is that aerobic exercise does help strengthen the cardiovascular and respiratory systems—that is, the heart and lungs—and that aerobic conditioning is important to general health, weight management and general quality of life. You won't be huffing and puffing every time you go about everyday activities that are a bit more demanding than usual.

Anaerobic exercise refers to muscle-building activities and fitness routines such as lifting weights that rely directly on oxygen for fuel. Since muscle burns more calories than fat, anaerobic activities indirectly contribute to weight management. The energy required for these relatively short but intense bursts of activity are fueled by non-oxygen sources stored in the muscles themselves. Because Nordic Walking is an upper-body workout as well as an aerobic activity, it is two for the price of one.

Another important benefit of using Nordic Walking poles is that the energy and exertion of the activity are transferred to more of the body, working the arms, shoulders, chest, and back as well as the legs and hips. Nordic Walking increases "core strength"—those muscles deep in the torso—that are important for maintaining health and vitality. Because the "burden" of the activity is shared by 90 percent of the body's muscle groups, Nordic Walkers often find that they can go faster and farther with poles than without poles—without having the feeling of a harder workout. If you have ever taken a step or other aerobics class, the instructor might have ended it with a pulse (or heart rate)

Donna Mirabile and Elizabeth Foote on Nordic Walking for Everyone

Plus-size Nordic Walkers Donna Mirabile and Elizabeth Foote were the subject of a Wall Street Journal story, have appeared on KSL-TV where they live in Salt Lake City, and, along with a sense of humor, have inspired out-of-shape people to get up and start moving. Tipping the scales at 300 pounds with health and mobility challenges, they both discovered Nordic Walking and what it could do for them.

Elizabeth Foote, who has type 2 diabetes, has been able to Nordic Walk although she is otherwise susceptible to exercise-induced asthma. She told a reporter from Salt Lake City's KSL-TV, "The first time I went Nordic Walking, I went out three times. My blood sugar dropped 20 points. So that got my attention. The fact my knees didn't hurt also got my attention. I could breathe and talk while I did this, and that got my attention too."

Donna Mirabile said, "My last blood pressure was 120 over 60, and my cholesterol went from 256 to 143." She has been certified as a LEKI Nordic Walking instructor. How inspiring she is for the overweight and out-of-shape! She continued, "In our experience, people who are very fit see fewer benefits from the poles than people who are not so fit. This is not to say that Nordic Walking does not benefit everyone, because it does. It just depends on what you are looking for.

"I think how much Nordic Walking raises the pulse depends upon the fitness level of the person doing it. For example, my pulse rises to a higher level sooner, and stays there more consistently, when I walk with my poles than when I use an elliptical trainer. Of course, I am 5 feet 8 inches tall, and eigh 340 pounds. My resting heart rate is 52.

"Being fat is no reason to go hide. I figure if people have a problem with how I look, they can look elsewhere! I love what I do with Nordic Walking and am convinced that it is the perfect exercise for people with chronic health problems like obesity and arthritis. I could go on and on about how I think the fitness industry fails people who are large.

"If someone wants to burn fat (which requires training at 40 and 60 percent of heart rate) and are very heavy, Nordic Walking is the perfect exercise. If someone just wants to burn fat and they're in decent shape, it's still a good choice. If someone wants to have a good cardio workout and they are not in shape enough to run, Nordic Walking is an excellent choice too. However, if someone is in good enough shape to run, they may need to either change the technique they use with Nordic Walking (i.e., do 'bounding' [which Nate Smith in Oregon was teaching] or some other method of using the poles) or as you mentioned, walking up a lot of hills.

Mirabile and Foote have formed FootePath, an enterprise designed to bring Nordic Walking to the less-active population who could benefit greatly, as they have, from physical activity. They offer Nordic Walking classes in the inspirational setting of the Olympic Oval, a legacy of Salt Lake City's 2002 Winter Olympic Games. This has the benefit of climate control and also enabling self-conscious new Nordic Walkers to take their first steps out of the public eye.

"My partner and I are targeting, the not so fit, as we spread the word about Nordic Walking," Mirabile notes. "We know from experience that people who have chronic illnesses that require them to exercise every day to be healthy often have no idea where to begin. Gyms can be intimidating. Also, when you exercise, insulin resistance is reduced in the body, but only in the muscles that are moving. Therefore, a full-body exercise that is gentle enough to be done every day, that doesn't hurt, and is fun is perfect."

check—or she might have asked you how hard you felt you worked —not very hard, medium hard or very hard.) A low perceived level of exertion translates to more bang for your exercise buck. If you don't feel that have exercised within your comfort zone, you can raise your intensity level without feeling that you have overworked.

Flexibility is also an important component of health and wellbeing, particularly as the body stiffens from lack of use or just from the passing of years. Regular practice of yoga, Pilates, Gyrotonics/Gyrokinesis or simply slow, gentle stretching is important for keeping the muscles from constricting and keeping the body limber and supple, which in turn contributes to overall well-being. Many Nordic Walking instruction programs begin with a short warm up routine that includes pre-walk stretching and finish with a cool-down that incorporates stretching which is particularly effective because warm, post-exercise muscles stretch more easily and farther than cool, pre-exercise ones.

Boning Up on Osteoporosis

Brittle bones. Dowager's hump. A broken hip. These are worrisome words for people as they age, most especially for post-menopausal women. In fact, women are four times more likely to contract osteoporosis than men, but men are hardly immune—and people who smoke or drink alcohol excessively are at increased risk compared to those who don't. This debilitating condition can affect virtually any bone in the body, but the hips, spine and wrists are particularly vulnerable. "Thin bones" become increasingly fragile and are more likely to break. If not prevented by weight-bearing exercise including Nordic Walking, sufficient calcium intake or medication, or if left untreated, osteoporosis can progress painlessly until a bone breaks.

The cure isn't pretty. Hip fractures generally require hospitalization including major surgery. In many cases, the patient's ability to walk unassisted is compromised forever. At its most serious, a broken hip can lead to prolonged or permanent disability, seriously diminishing the quality of life. Spinal or vertebral fractures lead to loss of height, severe back pain and crippling deformity. When you think about it, wouldn't you rather invest your time now exercising for the future payoff of a longer, more comfortable and healthier life?

In addition to adequate calcium intake (1,200 to 1,500 milligrams a day, plus vitamin D for absorption), women at risk are advised to do weight-bearing exercise to strengthen their bones. For those who also have joint problems, the same weight-bearing exercises that beef up the bones (running, walking, workouts with free weights or gym apparatus) can stress the joints. Again, that's when Nordic Walking is an exemplary exercise choice.

The underlying physiological reasons that exercise helps to maintain bone health can be explained quite simply. You know that muscles become bigger and stronger when you use them, because you can see them as they build. You can't see bones, but they also become stronger and denser when you place demands on them. There is a correlation between strong muscles and healthy bones. The complex biochemistry of muscle tugging on bones strengthens those bones. Exercising is good for both, and a lack of exercise, particularly as you age, may directly contribute to lower bone mass or density, as well as muscular weakness.

Nordic Walking is the perfect activity to combat osteoporosis, because it distributes the weight to both the upper and lower body. Therefore, it both relieves the leg joints from taking all the stress, while it also acts as a weight-bearing workout that strengthens the bones of the upper and lower body. At the same time, the joints are protected in ways that they are not in such other aerobic activities as jogging, running or even using a stair-stepper in a gym. Nordic Walking can help take

The Battle for Beautiful Bones

Here's what the National Osteoporosis Foundation has to say: "Just as a muscle gets stronger and bigger the more you use it, a bone becomes stronger and denser when you place demands on it.

"If your bones are not called upon to work, such as during physical activity, they do not receive any messages that they need to be strong. Thus, a lack of exercise, particularly as you get older, may contribute to lower bone mass or density.

You cannot see your bones respond to exercise, but when you strike a tennis ball or land on your feet after jumping, chemical messengers tell your arm and leg bones to be ready to handle that weight and impact again. In fact, if you x-ray the arms of a tennis player, you would see that the bones in the playing arm are bigger and denser than the bones in the other arm.

"Two types of exercises are important for building and maintaining bone mass and density: weight-bearing and resistance exercises. Weight-bearing exercises are those in which your bones and muscles work against gravity. This is any exercise in which your feet and legs are bearing your weight. Jogging, walking, stair climbing, dancing and soccer are examples of weight-bearing exercise with different degrees of impact. Swimming and bicycling are not weight bearing.

"The second type of exercises are resistance exercises or activities that use muscular strength to improve muscle mass and strengthen bone. These activities include weight lifting, such as using free weights and weight machines found at gyms and health clubs.

"Most weight-bearing and resistance exercises place health demands on bone. Daily activities and most sports involve a combination of these two types of exercises. Thus, an active lifestyle filled with varied physical activities strengthens muscles and improves bone strength."

"CAUTION: If you are frail, have had a fracture, fall frequently or have osteoporosis you should take extra caution. Certain movements like twisting of the spine, high impact aerobics or bending from the waist can be harmful. NOF recommends that before starting any exercise program, you should consult with a knowledgeable physician about your fracture risk."

the load off the knees and hips. By using poles when walking, you are decreasing the impact across the joint surface.

Because proper technique requires erect, upright carriage, Nordic Walkers often find that their posture improves. Nordic Walking also alleviates the tendency some people have toward favoring one side and becoming lopsided while walking without poles. The poling motion loosens the shoulders so that they are less inclined to hunch forward, and the spine straightens because standing erect feels better and more natural.

Pole Walking for Pain Relief

Even previously active people who develop painful joints often curtail their activity because it hurts too much. Arthritis can result in knee and hip pain that especially afflicts people who have subjected themselves to years of joint-pounding activities such as running (especially on pavement), high-impact aerobics, and mogul skiing. Studies have determined that Nordic Walking relieves up to 30 percent of the stress on the lower-body joints compared to walking without poles. Runners who train with poles can also significantly lessen joint stress and extend their pain-free running years. While years of running can cause pain, so can years of inactivity—and inactivity has been identified as a big risk factor for osteoarthritis. Unused muscles atrophy quickly and become unable to provide the structure and support that joints, especially knees, need. To get a sufficiently nourishing blood supply, cartilage in the knee requires the movement of muscle over bone.

Some back problems are really hip problems that manifest themselves in the lower back, so it is a good idea to work with a physiotherapist or other trained professional and to proceed cautiously when using Nordic Walking as a "cure" for back pain. Louise Kuebler, a New Zealand physiotherapist and Nordic Walking instructor, explains the difficulty that some people have under such conditions: "If a joint in your spine is inflamed, you feel stiff in the mornings, and pain occurs when the back gets stretched either in rotation or flexion. When the muscles are tight as well, Nordic walking actually aggravates your back pain, because it uses the already tight muscles at a strenuous level! I advise my patients to start Nordic Walking when the inflammation is subdued, mostly after four to six days." She advises stretching both before and after the walk and building up the length of the walk slowly. She also suggests using poles only three times a week to start.

Osteoarthritis is an umbrella word for a variety of disorders that lead to a joint's structural or functional failure. It affects the entire joint and also nearby muscles, underlying bone, ligaments, joint lining (synovium) and the joint cover (capsule). Further, it speeds up the loss of cartilage, which in turn causes the underlying bone to harden as the cartilage tries to repair itself. This "remodeled" bone plus the possible development of bone cysts eventually constrict and obliterate the natural space in the joint. Osteoarthritis has no easy cure, and other than pain medication, relief may come from surgery ranging from simple arthroscopy to joint replacement, but exercise can prevent or at least postpone such a procedure. Since contributing factors include obesity, diabetes and other endocrinological disorders and also post-injury conditions, doesn't it make sense to pick up a pair of poles and get moving as a preventive measure?

Advanced osteoarthritis is one excruciating form of chronic pain. According to the National Institute of Neurological Disorders and Stroke,

> "chronic pain persists. Pain signals keep firing in the nervous system for weeks, months, even years. There may have been an initial mishap—sprained back, serious infection, or there may be an ongoing cause of pain—arthritis, cancer, ear infection, but some people suffer chronic pain in the absence of any past injury or evidence of body damage. Many chronic pain conditions affect older adults. Common chronic pain complaints include headache, low back pain, cancer pain, arthritis pain, neurogenic pain (pain resulting from damage to the peripheral nerves or to the central nervous system itself), psychogenic pain (pain not due to past disease or injury or any visible sign of damage inside or outside the nervous system)."

Chronic pain is debilitating, even when there is no systemic or skeletal cause. For sufferers of common chronic aches and pains, including fibromyalgia, Nordic Walking often provides considerable relief. If you have undiagnosed aches, pain or stiffness, especially in such areas as the lower back, neck and shoulders, you will be surprised how much better you will feel if you begin Nordic Walking. A Finnish study conducted in 1999 by the Helsinki Polytechnic Stadia's Faculty of Health Care and Social Sciences investigated the link between

Cruel Shoes

Some forms of osteoarthritis are the result of choices we ourselves have made—especially "we" as in "WomEn." Shoe fashions that dictate, as they did in the '60s and again some four decades later, high spike heels and pointed toes are the precursors of a variety of complaints. Walking on very high heels is harmful to the feet, to the knees and to healthy body alignment, especially over a long period of time and even more so on hard pavement.

According to the American Society of Podiatric Sports Medicine, a 3-inch heel creates seven times more stress than a 1-inch heel, and those towering 4- and even 5-inchers are even worse, especially when they are narrow spikes. The American Academy of Orthopaedic Surgeons, whose members end up surgically correcting many of these self-inflicted problems counsels: no more than 3 hours in 3-inch heels.

Such high-heeled shoes result in more than just sore feet. They force the body and joints into unnatural positions, specifically creating excess pressure on the inside of the knees—a common site where women develop painful osteoarthritis. High heels also push the torso into an unnatural position, shifting the center of balance forward and throwing the spine and hips out of alignment. The higher the heel, the more pronounced these shifts are.

Additionally, women who wear "cruel shoes" all or most of the time may experience cramping of shortened calf muscles, tightened Achilles tendons, bunions, hammertoes, corns, calluses, pump bumps (thickened bone on the back of the heels), Morton's neuroma (toe pain and numbness caused by thickened tissue surrounding the nerve that runs between the third and fourth toes) and metatarsalgia (pain in the ball of the foot caused by body weight thrust forward because of high heels).

Nordic Walking can help alleviate these problems. So can buying good walking shoes and custom orthotics, and wearing those pricey *"Sex in the City"* shoes only on occasions when you will mostly be sitting down.

women who work mainly on computers, and their neck and shoulder problems as well as the mobility of their cervical and pectoral spines. Nordic Walking alleviated the neck and shoulder symptoms in more than half of the participants in the study. They also experienced significant improvements in mobility of the spine.

Hitting the Road to Everyday Fitness

Once you make Nordic Walking a part of your routine, take a step back and evaluate the rest of your life. Even conscientious Nordic Walkers don't get the maximum benefit from their new commitment to health and fitness if they alternate bursts of Nordic Walking activity with an otherwise sedentary and physically passive existence. The benefits of Nordic Walking are enhanced by developing daily habits of physical activity. Returning from an invigorating 30-minute Nordic Walk and flopping on the couch with the TV remote and a high-calorie snack may not totally defeat the purpose of the walk, but it certainly diminishes its effectiveness.

The AHA/ASA Start! program mentioned earlier is one of several national, regional and local motivational programs available to help people get moving and keep moving. The Cooper Institute's Active Living Every Day (ALED) philosophy is designed to introduce sedentary

The Cooper Institute's ALED program is based on research that produced these two important findings:
- Physical activity need not be strenuous or time-consuming to benefit health. Accumulating 30 minutes of moderate-intensity (e.g., a brisk walk) activity on most days of the week can result in significant health benefits.
- People are more likely to become and stay physically active when taught appropriate lifestyle skills. These skills include identifying and overcoming barriers to physical activity, learning to fit physical activity into a busy schedule, increasing self-confidence, building social support, setting realistic goals, and staying motivated.

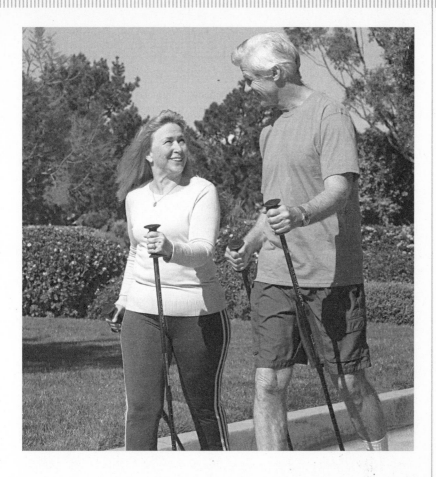

people to skills that will help them become and stay physically active for a lifetime, such as overcoming barriers to physical activity, realistic goal setting, building confidence and staying motivated.

Nordic Walking and Issues Affecting the Elderly

As people grow older, as we all eventually expect to, balance and stability are impacted—and because the consequences of falls can be greater, people tend to be afraid to move just when they should try to maintain their agility. The issue of osteoporosis was addressed above, but it bears repeating. Nordic Walking poles amount to a pair of tubular security blankets. Nordic Walkers have four on the floor, not just two, which helps balance and improves confidence to get moving and keep moving.

Aging can also affect the mind. An aging population means a dramatic increase in dementia, Alzheimer's disease and other cognitive problems that affect the elderly.

According to the Fisher Center for Alzheimer's Disease Foundation,

"Maintaining a reasonable level of exercise is important for many reasons, both for overall health and to address issues specific to Alzheimer's. Exercise can improve mobility and help one maintain independence. In normal people, moderately strenuous exercise has been shown to improve cognitive functioning. In people with Alzheimer's, studies show that light exercise and walking appear to reduce wandering, aggression and agitation. Incorporating exercise into daily routines and scheduled activities can also be beneficial in alleviating problem behaviors. The type of exercise should be individualized to the person's abilities. Talk with your doctor about what is right."

Child-development authorities have long known that the motor skill of crawling and walking—with limbs in opposition, (left leg/right hand, right leg/left arm)—helps cognitive development. Some people similarly believe that the oppositional movements of Nordic Walking can help seniors retain their mental acuity and perhaps also curtail deterioration of brain function. "Any activity that uses cross-flexor and cross-extensor movements and reflex activity supports whole-brain integration," notes Paul Chek of the C.H.E.K. Institute, a leader in fitness education.

"Use it or lose it." We all have heard the phrase. This is especially true for older people who slow down and become increasingly less active—either due to illness, injury or just the natural aging process —and therefore continue to lose mobility, strength and independence. Nordic Walking is no total fountain of youth, but it does show real promise in enabling the elderly to keep on using it so that they won't lose it. Peggy Buchanan, named 1997 Fitness Instructor of the Year and spokesperson on older adult fitness, conducted the first 8-week pilot study with 13 subjects averaging 87 years of age. This group, although small, put aside their canes and walkers and picked up Exerstrider fitness-walking poles. Buchanan observed, "People with canes and walkers tend to see themselves as 'invalids,' but the same people with walking poles more often feel like 'athletes.' Those who traded in both walkers and canes immediately began walking with a

Fitness Poles for the Super-Seniors

To address the needs of the growing elderly market, Exerstrider in 2007 introduced the Activator Medisport Edition, the first adjustable-length pole since the company was established in 1988. This pole utilizes the same type of "snap button/hole length adjustment" mechanism commonly used on canes and walkers. Physical therapists are familiar with it, and people with limited hand strength can manage it. Other features familiar to Exerstrider users are the strapless/safety ergonomic grips and boot-shaped Cushiongrip rubber paws. There is also an optional bell-shaped balance tip for people with balance issues or who just feel more comfortable with that shape.

more upright posture and their gait pattern went from a 'shuffle' to a more normal walking gait."

She also noted, "The psychological benefits may have been just as important as the physical benefits." Using walking poles can aid in providing balance, confidence and relief for painful joints, and at the same time, they can also help build upper-body muscles and aid in preventing bone loss, as walking becomes a total-body, weight-bearing activity." As a result, Nordic Walkers have an increased self-image, and because Nordic Walking is fun and also feels secure, pole users tend to remain more active, which in turn makes them stronger and more agile—and all that jazz.

Nordic Walking for People with Disabilities

While many conditions, such as osteoporosis, can be prevented or mitigated, others cannot be—at least not at this writing and not for most people. Nordic Walking is suitable for some people with multiple sclerosis, Parkinson's and other motor-neurological disorders, as well

Nancy Deals with Dementia Through Nordic Walking

In a piece called "Living in Mind" published in the *Highlands News*, Scottish writer Margaret Chrystall, wrote about Nancy, who "spends her spring and summer days working in her big garden, she dances, goes to exercise class, enjoys Nordic Walking and camping. In her early sixties, Nancy believes in getting the most out of her life—and for the last few years, that has meant living with dementia. It's a condition that...hit the headlines with the release of a new, much-praised film, *Away From Her*, where Julie Christie plays a woman coming to terms with the changes dementia brings to her life."

Nancy exercises her body and her mind, both in a regular gym and in a "brain gym" that, among other things, "makes connections" between the right and left sides of the brain. "I also do Nordic Walking for an hour once a week," Nancy told the reporter. "You use skiing sticks to help you walk and you can get up quite a speed. It makes you feel very powerful."

as some amputees. Obviously if you have an illness or other medical condition, the caution to "check with your doctor" is even more important than for healthy but out-of-shape beginners. It might be necessary to work with a physical therapist or with a Nordic Walking instructor who is keyed into and trained for these special situations.

You might consider Reinhild Moeller of Incline Village NV, to be such a person. She was only 3½ years old when she became a below-the-knee amputee after an accident on the family farm in southern Germany. When her parents were bringing in grain, the toddler fell under the harvester. Her parents, she says, were devastated, "But it was a godsend for me." Her disability challenged her to excel in sports. A natural athlete, she became a ski racer who competed for her native Germany in the Paralympics, winning gold and silver medals; she was a sprinter and long-jumper in the Summer Games, and even competed against able-bodied cyclists in mountain bike competitions. Along the way, she earned a master's degree in sports science and adaptive physical education.

Nordic Walking, which she discovered on one of her trips to Germany, opened another frontier for her. "When I first saw people doing it, I thought that it should be a sport," Moeller said. "And I figured that Lake Tahoe would be the perfect place to do it. We've got trails and a lot of people who are really into physical health."

Her husband, Reed Robinson, an arm amputee and also a Paralympic ski champion, was always the stronger hiker. "I brought poles back from Germany," Moeller says. "It was amazing how well I could keep up with him. With a below-the-knee amputation, I could never push off as much, and there was also the issue of balance." Poles, she believes, can help "any leg amputee," though Robinson told her, "This isn't a sport for me." Nordic Walking certainly doesn't meet the requirements of all disabilities, but it can help people a surprising number of different physical challenges.

Michelle Honer on Nordic Walking Poles to Combat Chronic Disability

Multiple sclerosis was no obstacle to Nordic Walking, reports Pete Edwards, pole-walking advocate and founder of skiwalking.com.

"While hosting Nordic Walking at The Fitness Center in Traverse City, Michigan, I was introduced to Michelle Honer. Michelle had signed up to participate in one of my Ski Walking classes. When she walked up the handicap ramp prior to the class with her cane, it was apparent that she had some balance issues. She informed her classmates that she had MS. Our first Ski Walk was only a few blocks down and back. Within several weeks, we were covering about 2 miles in 1 hour.

"For 7 prior years, Michelle had ridden an electric scooter in the Traverse City MS Walk. The last couple years, Michelle has Ski Walked the 5K (3.1 miles). Local newspapers and TV stations have covered her remarkable story.

"'My special Nordic Walking poles have allowed me to walk taller, faster, further and with much more stability than with my cane. Their one-piece design is so much better than my old adjustable poles that broke unexpectedly at an extremely inconvenient time,' says Michelle.

"Michelle is now an official Ski Walking Ambassador for skiwalking.com and proudly wears her Ski Walking shirt made of organic cotton while assisting at many of my Nordic Walking Clinics.

"Michelle's success with the walking poles encouraged me to host free Nordic Walking Clinics at MS support group meetings. She suggested that I also contact the Jimmie Heuga Center in Colorado. The Heuga Center is dedicated to helping those with MS lead healthier and happier lives."

– told by Pete Edwards, founder of skiwalking.com, developer of the American Nordic Walking System and US distributor of Swix Nordic Walking poles.

Author's Note: Colorado's Heuga Center for Multiple Sclerosis was founded by Jimmie Heuga, an Olympic skiing medal winner who contracted MS. As an athlete, he was not content to sit down and rest, as doctors advised when he was diagnosed. His approach was to remain as active as his condition permitted at any time.

The Heuga Center has adopted his philosophy. Its programs, services and events reinforce a positive attitude for people coping with the disease. "We believe that every person diagnosed with multiple sclerosis deserves the opportunity to maintain their overall health and well-being so that they may live the most productive, fulfilling life possible.

"We believe that MS affects the entire family; that knowledge is power; that physical and emotional fitness is key; and that a positive, 'can do' attitude is the most fruitful approach to managing this chronic, unpredictable disease."

Gini Patterson, physical therapist and chair of the Heuga Center's Board of Directors, confirms, "Nordic walking is a great way for people with multiple sclerosis to improve their aerobic capacity while at the same time build some upper body strength. The lightweight poles increase your base of support for those individuals who may have some balance challenges."

Pregnancy and Post-Partum Exercise

Barring complications or special medical considerations, most doctors now recommend that women keep active during their pregnancies in order to stay healthier, fitter and more energetic and also to have easier deliveries. Nordic Walking again fits right in with these recommendations. Because it is a low-impact, total-body workout that can be done at whatever speed is comfortable, it is a suitable exercise, often well into the third trimester. As a woman's center of gravity changes, poles offer the additional benefit of security and lessen the chance of stumbling or falling. A physicians' association in Germany specifically recommends it as one way to lessen the likelihood of developing varicose veins during pregnancy. Nordic Walking is the gift that keeps on giving before and after childbirth. A new mother can get back to it after the baby is born, as soon as the doctor approves. New moms can pick up their poles and start walking again to start feeling "normal" again and to speed the shedding of pregnancy pounds. Some women welcome the opportunity to leave the baby with Dad while they Nordic Walk, while others wouldn't dream of doing that. Small infants can be brought along in benign weather, in a forward-facing carrier and later in a backpack-style carrier. Both leave the hands free for poles. Because Nordic Walking can be done anywhere, exercise time is flexible, and in most cases, it isn't necessary to go far from home. All an expectant or new mom needs to do is step out the door, find a clear path or sidewalk or a quiet roadway suitable for Nordic Walking and get moving.

Moderate Exercise Can Combat Depression

Regular exercise, fresh air and sunshine (or at least daylight) are anecdotally known to lift the spirits, and science is backing up conventional wisdom on the matter. Several studies show that regular, moderate exercise is at least as effective in combating even clinical depression as popular prescription drugs and preventing the condition from returning. "A lot of people know from their own experience that when they exercise, they feel better," concluded James A. Blumenthal, professor of psychology at Duke University and lead researcher on studies examining the impact of exercise versus antidepressant drugs in combating depression. Both anecdotal and placebo-controlled clinical trials came to the same conclusion. The first Duke study involved 156 adults who volunteered for a 4-month comparison of exercise alone, a brand-name antidepressant alone and a combination of exercise and medication. The exercise was moderate: just 30 minutes, plus warm up and cool-down, three times a week. In that study, published in 2000, patients in all groups had comparable improvements, with about 60 percent of the exercisers reporting vastly improved or no symptoms of depression, compared with about 66 percent of the group on medication and 69 percent of the combination group. Patients in all groups had comparable improvements, the researchers said. Even moderate exercise turns out to be the gift that keeps on giving. About 60 percent of the exercisers vastly improved or had no symptoms, compared with about 66 percent of the medication group and 69 percent of the combination group. In a controlled follow-up study of 202 patients published in 2007, Blumenthal reported that after 16 weeks, 47 percent of those who took the antidepressant drug improved, as did 45 percent of those who exercised in supervised groups and 40 percent of those who exercised on their own. About 30 percent in the placebo group improved. The statistical difference between the exercise and medication groups is not considered major.

Start 'Em Young, Keep 'Em Fit

Childhood obesity, like obesity in the general population, has come to be called an "epidemic." The statistics are staggering—and frightening—because obese children have juvenile health risks, including the dreaded childhood diabetes. Even if they manage to be overweight yet healthy while they are growing up, obese youngsters tend to become obese adults with all the problems that implies. According to the Centers for Disease Control and the National Association for Sport and Physical Education, between 5 and 6.5 percent of all American youngsters were overweight 20 years ago. Today, 17.4 percent of those ranging in age from 12 to 19, 18.8 percent of children ages 6 to 11 and a staggering 13.9 percent of preschoolers ages 2 to 5 are overweight. Much media attention has been cast on the causes—the relentless consumption of too much junk food, too much time in front of the television or playing video games, the cutback in physical education in school systems across the land, too little parental trust that children can safely walk or ride their bikes to school and other causes that are beyond the scope of this book.

Even sedentary-by-choice children have innate youthful energy, and if they don't run it off at play, they often start getting restless in class. They fidget and their minds wander and many—mostly boys—are then diagnosed with attention deficit disorder. The solution? Often medication—but isn't exercise, which used to be called "letting off steam," a better way to help children settle down and pay attention in class?

Experts are also finding this to be true. According to Dawn Coe, lead researcher in a study conducted at Michigan's Grand Valley State University, "Physical activity may reduce boredom and increase attention span and concentration. Increased activity levels may lead to higher levels of self-esteem. And all of these factors may play a role in the relationship between physical activity and academic performance." The study indicated that as little as 20 minutes of vigorous physical activity just three times a week can help academic performance.

Eating disorders developed in a misguided effort to become very thin are an epidemic of another sort. Many little girls want to look like their Barbie dolls, and as they get older, they want to look like emaciated celebrities. The average American woman is 5 feet, 4 inches tall and weighs 140 pounds. The average fashion model is 5 feet, 11 inches tall and weighs 117 pounds. Girls—and it is mostly adolescent girls and young women—do terrible things to their bodies and their health in order to try to reach this impossible, and in truth undesirable, goal. These include anorexia, bulimia and eating disorders and other unhealthy behaviors. Calorie-burning physical activity is not always part of the adolescent weight-loss game plan, but it should be. The result of these poor choices is a generation populated by too many malnourished, reed-thin young females who do nothing to keep their bones and muscles strong. This, of course, also lays the groundwork for unhealthy adulthood, including—but not limited to—fertility issues.

Just as overweight adults are more likely to be injured than those of normal weight, overweight children and adolescents are more likely to suffer bone fractures, and even joint and muscle pain, than their normal-weight peers, according to a study of youngsters in Washington, DC, conducted at the National Institutes of Health. Of the 355 youngsters, both black and white, 227 were classified as overweight; 128 not. If not dealt with, youngsters' weight problems of can linger into adulthood. Overweight but growing youngsters were also more likely to develop knee problems. For example, 21.4 percent of the overweight children already were reporting knee pain. "Bone, muscle and joint problems are particularly troubling in this age group," said Dr. Elias A. Zerhouni, NIH Director. "If overweight youth fail to attain normal weight, they will likely experience an even greater incidence of these problems when they reach later life."

Hand a kid a pair of Nordic Walking poles, and watch the fun begin. Youngsters often break out into spontaneous "Nordic Skipping" or "Nordic Bounding," often running circles around their parents if the family is going out together. Technique doesn't matter nearly as much as the sheer joy and the healthy exercise. Some companies, notably Exel and LEKI, make or have made children's Nordic Walking poles. Adjustable poles that grow as the child does are a good solution to the what-size-to-issue decision.

Tim "T-Bone" Arem on Children and Nordic Walking

"T-Bone" provides real insight into how Nordic Walking can fit into the promotion of healthy activity for the nation's children. He is an enthusiastic fitness ambassador who has created an elementary school program to make that happen. Arem sees a "natural link between youth health and fitness and Nordic Walking," not surprising for a man with a master's degree in education, a gift for entertaining children and a natural affinity for making fitness fun. In the past, he had gigs portraying such kid-pleasing characters as Ronald McDonald, Mac Tonight and one of the Teenage Mutant Ninja Turtles, but after promoting unhealthy fast food, he is making up for it by encouraging kids to become healthy, fast-moving and fit. To that end, he developed T-Bone, a costumed character who shares the benefits of children's health and physical fitness.

He says that he connects with tens of thousands of families, both in schools and at running events where he puts on a pre-race warm up and entertaining act called "T-Bone's Magic and Fitness Adventure." He is also such a Nordic Walking nut that he even published a small book about it. *Nordic Walking: A Total Body Experience* addresses fitness issues for all ages, but it is regarding children that he makes his message clearest.

"My mission is health and fitness from youth to adulthood," he says. "With so many exciting things in our culture like computers, video games and TV, it's definitely a fun challenge to teach kids about the importance of eating right and staying fit. I really believe the message is getting out there. I'm asked back year after year to more than 40 different races a year."

"Of the 100,000 children I work with in schools, 30 to 40 percent maintain a life of little fitness activity," he says, adding, "I have chosen a positive approach to teaching Nordic Walking in schools to give less-active children a fun way to incorporate healthy activity into their lives. A very cool thing that I hear from teachers who I work with is that active children find Nordic Walking interesting. When less-active, less-fit children see their peers doing this activity, they want to participate too." For the 2006/2007 school year, T-Bone Productions introduced Nordic Walking Across America (NWAA), a national initiative for elementary schools to encourage kids to be active.

"My goal," Arem says, "is to provide fun, interactive, healthy ways to install healthy habits into our nation's children. As we all are aware, we often take into adulthood what we learn in our youth. Nordic Walking is an awesome tool to share with our children and families."

Conventional wisdom used to be that an ounce of prevention is worth a pound of cure. It still is, so consider Nordic Walking to be part of the ounce of prevention to ward off any number of ailments in adults and children alike, and to mitigate the effects of many illnesses or chronic conditions, once contracted.

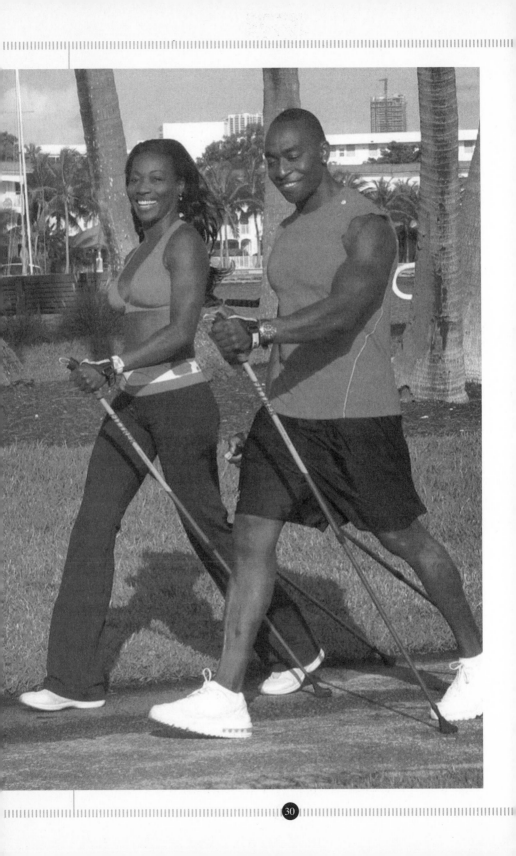

Gearing Up:
Nordic Walking
Poles

Nordic Walking doesn't require much in the way of equipment other than specially designed, lightweight poles and good, sturdy footwear. You might want to use walking or running shoes that you already own, especially when you begin and aren't ready to make a major investment in new footwear. Once you hit your stride, literally and figuratively, it's time to consider shoes that are designed specifically for Nordic Walking. One caveat is that no matter how dedicated you become, you might find it difficult to buy new shoes designed for this new sport. In that case, good-quality walking shoes or trail running shoes are your best bet. In addition to poles, footwear and suitable clothing make Nordic Walking comfortable, and once you get hooked, you'll find an assortment of optional accessories to make your walks more efficient or pleasurable.

(Footwear is covered extensively in Chapter 3 and accessories in Chapter 4.)

Poles, however, are another matter. You need them right away because, obviously, you can't go Nordic Walking without them. Old ski poles won't do. In fact, not even cross-country ski poles will do. Hiking and trekking poles aren't really right either. Forgive the pun, but proper poles and unsuitable poles are poles apart. No matter what else is said about Nordic Walking, and no matter which name you use, it is always identified as a form of walking with poles. When you see someone Nordic Walking, those poles are immediately obvious, even from a distance. And when you begin the sport yourself, how, where and when you touch the pole tips to the ground during your stride is the first thing you learn.

Many beginner-level Nordic Walking classes and some group outings include the use of poles during the program. Others offer participants the opportunity to rent them inexpensively during the class. And in many cases, instructors offer the poles available during the program, perhaps at a discounted price. As more businesses get into Nordic Walking, you will probably find rental poles readily available in many places. They are widely available in European resorts and hopefully will be in North America when demand increases.

At first glance, it might seem as if Nordic Walking poles and trekking poles are the same. However, their form and their function are both different. Trekking poles are used by hikers for support, balance and stability, as well as to ease walking on uneven, rocky and/or steep ground, even when carrying a heavy backpack. Nordic Walking poles, by contrast, are designed for propulsion on relatively even and often smooth ground. Nordic Walking pole shafts are therefore thinner and lighter than trekking poles and in that regard, resemble cross-country ski poles. The poles' weight, swing weight and balance are important comfort factors when Nordic Walking, especially on a long walk.

At this writing, the retail price range for Nordic Walking poles is from about $50 for a bargain on a basic one-piece model to about $200 for a brand-name adjustable model made of high-grade materials. Replacement grips, straps, tips and paws—all discussed below—are available.

Anatomy of Nordic Walking Poles

The lightweight, tapered and yet sturdy **pole shafts** made for Nordic Walking can be of various materials. The three most common are carbon (or carbon-fiber), composite and aluminum alloy. **Carbon-fiber** is a strong, lightweight resin material made by heat-treating rayon or other synthetic fiber. In addition to being lightweight, it is known for its inherent vibration-damping properties. Some manufacturers use the same fabrication and materials for all of their pole shafts, while others make higher-priced and lower-priced ones differently. **Composite** pole shafts are made of resin and fiberglass, with or without a carbon-fiber component. **Aluminum alloys** are made of strong, lightweight metal. Some poles combine two kinds of materials—for example, aluminum on the top end of the shaft and a synthetic on the bottom.

Most pairs of Nordic Walking poles come with specific right- and left-hand poles, not because of the shaft but because of the pole grips—(the "handles" that you grasp when walking.) Make sure you

LEKI

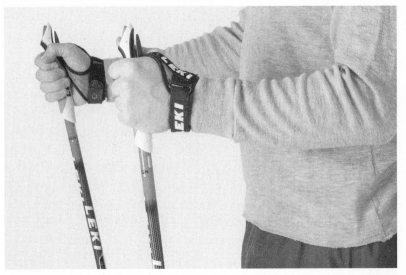

EXERSTRIDER

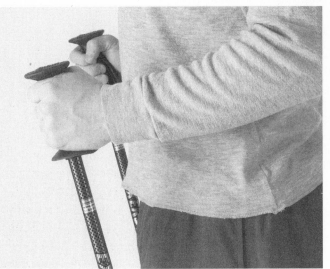

get a matching pair of poles, not a set of twins. The grips may be synthetic or cork. Because cork does not conduct heat or cold, many people find this material to be more comfortable in very hot or very cold weather.

While ski and trekking pole grips are roughly round and are always linear continuations of the straight shafts, most Nordic Walking pole grips are ergonomically oval and often slightly tilted, tipping back and perhaps also in toward the body. These subtle angles are more comfortable and natural for the wrists and hands. Because Exerstrider is a strapless pole, the bottom of the grip features a protruding flange to support the heel of the hand during the push-off phase.

Unlike trekking poles' or ski poles' simple, fairly narrow woven wrist straps, most Nordic Walking poles have thicker, cushioned **straps** that have been likened to fingerless gloves. Because Nordic Walking technique calls for a firm pole plant at the beginning of each poling motion and a comfortably open hand at the apex of what might be thought of as the backswing (the end of each poling motion), wide, comfortable straps provide support during the pole plant at the beginning of each stride and allow just control of the pole at the end, even though the hand is open. Equally importantly, these wide straps are cushioned to protect the heel of the hand to relieve the pressure created by planting the pole. Manufacturers often make them in several sizes, but within each size range, they are also adjustable via Velcro or a slide-buckle. That combination covers the range from small, gloveless hands to large gloved ones. Fittrek's Quick-Switch straps are interchangeable to accommodate different uses without having to buy two or three different pairs poles.

Most straps are affixed to the pole **grips**, though a few (currently Boomyah, Iwalk2, Joy, LEKI, Nordixx and optional straps on several smaller brands)

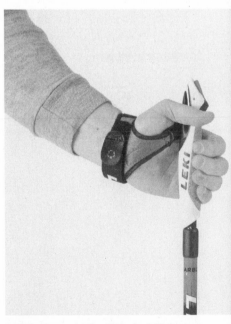

LEKI strap with click-in/click-out feature

have some kind of a click-in/click-out feature, so you can release the poles quickly to use your hands without extracting them from the straps. This is useful for, say, retying a shoelace or unwrapping a snack bar. If you want to reapply sunscreen, however, you probably ought to remove the straps so you don't goop them up. Exerstrider, the exception, uses strapless grips for reasons given in the brand rundown below.

A slightly blunted metal **tip** or spike, usually made of carbide, tungsten or steel at the base (bottom) of each pole shaft is intended for off-pavement walking. These metal tips are often also angled to continue the efficient transfer of power from the grips through the shafts to the ground. Bare tips are best used when the walking surface is dirt, gravel or hard sand, or for snowshoeing in winter.

Some kind of a rubber **paws** (also called **caps**, **feet**, **booties** or **boots**) slip over the tips and fit firmly for use when walking on pavement or for storage or transport. They come in various styles from round or bell-shaped rubber paws to splayed, foot-like designs. When they are shaped like paws, the "toes" are designed to point backwards. LEKI also makes a studded rubber cap that offers additional traction on ice or hard snow. Combine them with under-boot traction devices, and winter-slick surfaces are no reason not to go Nordic Walking in winter.

While the shafts and metal tips on quality poles last a really long time, paws eventually do wear out. Pole manufacturers make replacements. How often they need to be replaced depends on how much you use them and how aggressively you push off with each stride—and of course, the quality of the material. Consider 6 months as a ballpark for the life of a pair of rubber paws

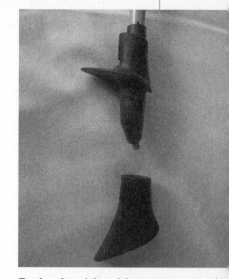

Exel pole with rubber paw

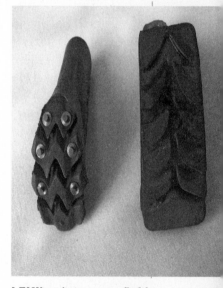

LEKI's winter paw (left) and all-season paw (right)

if you use them several times a week and generally walk on pavement. Some people, especially those who live in such rainy places as the coastal areas of northern California, Washington, Oregon and British Columbia, believe that one style or even one brand is better than others in providing traction on wet, slick pavement. Larger paws with bigger footprints offer better traction, just like wider tires on a car or bicycle. Instead of removable paws, Swix poles feature a distinctive hinged mechanism attached to the poles that can be flicked between metal tip and rubber foot, and Joy poles, a brand currently available only in Europe, can be switched from metal tip to rubber paw with a quick twist. Each type has its advantages. Attached caps cannot easily be lost or misplaced, while removable ones are easier to replace when they wear out. It is not necessary for replacement paws to be the same brand as the poles. They are interchangeable, as long as the diameter of the pole shaft matches the diameter of the hole in the paw.

The final chapter on Nordic Walking poles has not been written. As the activity grows in popularity, modifications and innovations are continuously being made. Exerstrider's Activator Medisport Edition became the first pole to incorporate the same kind of snap button/hole length adjustment mechanism commonly used on canes and walkers. It is easier for people who have been using walking aids, physical therapists and caregivers to use. The length of Boomyah poles can be easily and intuitively adjusted. A pair of Gymstick walking poles can be coupled together to become a single pole that incorporates resistance bands. Amy Cheryl, a former bodybuilder, trainer and creator of Flexxation Sculpting Systems of Los Angeles, takes classes hiking up one of the canyons off the Pacific Coast Highway. She finds a suitable spot for her class to do the sculpting part of the workout. "L.A. is a big outdoorsy place," she says. "Combining a hike and sculpting is impressive and effective. With Gymstick, you don't need to bring any other products on your walk for a complete workout."

Two Tips on Tips

- If you find that the caps or paws wear down unevenly, it might be because you are pushing off more aggressively on one side than the other. The "cure" can focus on training yourself to push of evenly on both sides – unless the unevenness is physical and cannot be corrected. If that is the case, change the paws from one pole to another periodically so that they wear down at about the same time.

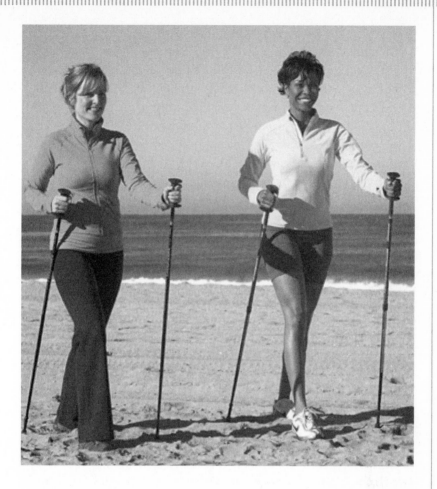

- Pulling the rubber paws off the tips can take a fair amount of strength, especially when you have been pressuring them with every strike, when grit has come between rubber and metal, or when a vacuum has developed under the paw. If you think of it in advance, put a little baby powder into the paw before fitting it over the tip. Otherwise, use your feet. Squeeze the rubber tip between the inside edges of your shoe soles, either just at the ball of the foot or where your big toes join your forefoot. Press your feet together to pressure the paw while you tug on the pole shaft.

   Pole baskets—discs with a hole in the center that slip over the tips of the bottom few inches of the poles—are useful for Nordic Walking on sand and snow (and also snowshoeing). Komperdell is an example of a brand with integrated cushioning paws and small baskets, but most are removable and prevent the tip from sinking into sand or in snow when snowshoeing.

The difference between **fixed length** and **adjustable poles** is obvious just from the names. Fixed-length poles (also called one-piece poles) have one-piece shafts and are lighterweight than adjustable poles made of the same materials because there is no mechanism in the shafts. Adjustable poles have telescoping shafts and can be lengthened or shortened by twisting them in one direction to loosen and release and the other direction to tighten and lock—or occasionally by snapping them.

Some new Nordic Walkers simply buy the poles sold by their instructors, often at a discount. They have become accustomed to the poles with which they took their first Nordic Walking steps and the feel of the grips and straps is so comfortable that they are content to stick with them. Other people try both types of poles—and perhaps different brands—as a basis for deciding which kind to buy. And some Nordic Walkers eventually have at least one pair of each.

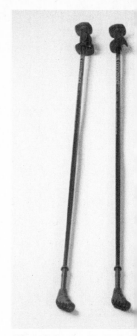

Fixed-Length Poles

Benefits of One-Piece (Fixed-Length) Poles

One-piece poles usually come in 5-centimeter increments, often from 100 to 140 centimeters. Some Nordic Walkers prefer the balance or swing weight of one-piece poles, and some also like the fact that they are quieter during the walk. If you select this type, remember the importance of buying the correct length—and that in itself is a little tricky because some people find it more comfortable to learn with shorter poles and "graduate" to longer ones when they become proficient. Another advantage of one-piece poles is that there is no adjustment mechanism to wear out if the length is changed frequently and perhaps with too much force. Some Nordic Walkers have found that the mechanism in inexpensive adjustable poles breaks down sooner than they expected.

Benefits of Adjustable (Telescoping) Poles

A mechanism within the shafts of adjustable poles enables the user to loosen the pole, change its length and tighten it again. These poles are made in two or occasionally three sections and twist to adjust, with a locking mechanism to keep them at the desired length. Because people of different heights can easily share adjustable poles, they are popular in Nordic Walking classes. Some people also prefer slightly longer poles as they improve, because they find longer poles to provide a better workout. Adjustable poles are also good for growing youngsters. People who frequently walk up and down steep hills often prefer adjustable poles, because they can be lengthened on downhills, shortened on uphills and set for the length that would be proper for a fixed-length pole on the flats. Adjustable poles also can be collapsed to fit into a suitcase or duffel bag for travel.

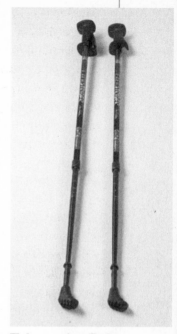

Telescoping Poles

The Debate: One-Piece or Adjustable

For some Nordic Walkers, the choice of one-piece or adjustable is clear from the outset. For others, it is simply a matter of taste often related to which kind they first used. For still others—mostly instructors or others in the Nordic Walking business—the choice is practically a moral issue with "right" and "wrong" types of poles. Proponents of one-piece poles complain that adjustables sometimes collapse while in use. People who prefer adjustables note that if and when they want a longer pole as they get better, they have to buy another pair. The debate continues. Manufacturers sometimes compromise with partially adjustable poles that don't collapse fully but can be fine-tuned within about a 10-centimeter range. Sheri Simson, a self-described Nordic Walking and fitness ambassador in Canada who developed the Keenfit pole, makes another case for adjustable poles. She says that most people don't ever tinker with the length once they've found one that they like, but in principle, she says that they like this micro-adjustability. She notes that even people who measure the same on a height chart are built differently. Short or long torsos, short or long legs, and short or long arms can affect correct pole use, and only when a person has gotten into Nordic Walking can the most suitable length be determined.

SkiWalking founder Pete Edwards is an equally passionate advocate for lighterweight, quieter one-piece poles. He points out that "skiers don't use adjustable/telescoping/adjustable poles and neither should" Nordic Walkers. He contends that that "adjustable poles vibrate and rattle, especially on pavement and other hard surfaces," and he also has said that "hundreds of backpackers have tumbled down the trail when their telescoping poles unexpectedly collapsed, causing serious injury." Hundreds? All backpackers (which implies use of a trekking pole) and all of them seriously injured? That was a pretty dramatic statement—one that he began to back away from. Still, the fervor and frequency with which he states it speaks to the strength of his belief. In any case, adjustable poles *can* collapse, causing annoyance and frustration, if not injury. The non-secret secret is to tighten them enough so that they don't loosen when pressured but not so tightly that you need a wrench to loosen them. Another solution is Boomyah's unique click-closure, which does not involve rotating the two parts of the shaft to lock and unlock.

The bottom line is that every Nordic Walker contemplating a pole purchase needs to decide for himself or herself which is the better choice—one-piece or adjustable poles, or perhaps a pair of each.

Sheri Simson on Becoming a Nordic Walking Entrepreneur

Sheri Simson is a 40-plus housewife, mother and business owner who not only talks the talk, but walks the walk— literally. After she discovered Nordic Walking on a trip to Europe, she became an advocate and established her own pole company, Keenfit of Kelowna, British Columbia. She also leads Nordic Walking group sessions and is positively messianic about the weight-loss and toning benefits of the sport:

"As the owner of my own successful construction company, wife and mother of three boys (the oldest 7 and the youngest just about to turn 2), finding time to exercise, eat healthy and relax seemed impossible. Carrying three babies full term had done a number on my body and

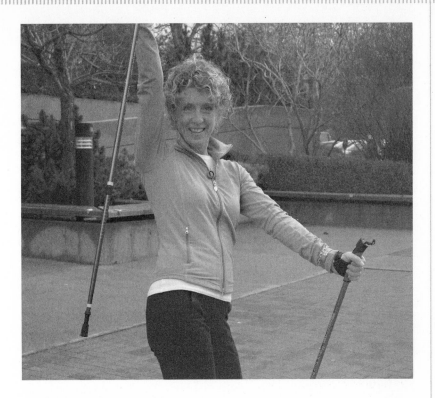

my back, and I had held onto a few extra pounds with each pregnancy. I not only felt unattractive, but I was tired all the time.

"I was 41, 30 pounds overweight and terribly out of shape. My once fairly fit, strong body was far from it. I had extra skin and fat, weak, limp muscles, and cellulite in places I never knew you could get cellulite. And I had aches and pains all over, not just here and there. Never would I dare be seen in anything sleeveless, and for years, I felt embarrassed if anyone but my family saw me in a bathing suit. I blamed a lot of it on the fact that I was over 40.

"Desperate, I signed up for Weight Watchers and realized that, though I thought I was eating well, I was—but just a little too well! Weight Watchers really helped me change the way I look at food and how I approach eating. I don't diet. I just watch what I eat!

"I finally started going in the right direction. I was watching what I was eating and I was starting to lose weight, but I still felt sluggish, tired and out of shape. With juggling my full-time business and busy family I had little time, energy or extra money to get into shape. Walking was all I had the time or money for, but just walking seemed to have little effect on how I looked and felt.

"It was a trip to Europe that introduced me to fitness-walking and Nordic Walking. I brought home a pair of walking poles. I was excited to put them to work and was blown away by the results they produced. It was so easy that at first I thought it was maybe too easy—no pain pain, no gain. But once I got a rhythm going, my whole body felt almost energized, as the poles seemed to propel me forward.

"It truly didn't take long for me to notice a difference between walking without poles and walking with them. My fat just fell off, and within weeks, I felt stronger and definitely tighter. It was amazing. The funny thing was I wasn't walking any further or any faster. I couldn't get over what was happening to what seemed to be every inch of my body. And I had so much more energy, not to mention experiencing and watching my body take on its new shape helped me feel so much better about myself. For the first time in a long time, I actually felt sexy. I had arms like Madonna, and I wasn't even lifting weights.

"I made it my mission to raise the fitness level of North America—one stride at a time. It was not long ago that I, like many North Americans, was too busy, overweight and exhausted —or so I thought. So why not allow everyone who walks to enjoy the amazing benefits of this fun, simple, full-body exercise? "

Buying or Setting the Correct Length

If you opt for adjustable poles, skip a few paragraphs, but if you are buying one-piece, fixed-length poles, you need to get the correct length. Poles are made in 5-centimeter (about 2-inch) increments. If you go to a brick-and-mortar store for your Nordic Walking poles, you will be asked to stand in your walking shoes and place your hands in the pole straps. If your forearms are parallel to the floor, you have found the proper length.

If you are ordering online, you need to do some calculation, unless you find a Web site that does it for you. The standard formula is to multiply your height (in centimeters) by roughly 65 percent. If the figure falls between two standard pole lengths, most experts recommend rounding down. There are some tweaks to these formulas too. Some experts believe in subtracting two inches from that number. Nordic Pole Walking, which carries Nordixx poles, recommends the length that enables the forearm to be parallel to the floor for "active" or advanced Nordic Walkers and two inches shorter for recreational or "wellness" walkers. Fittrek and others

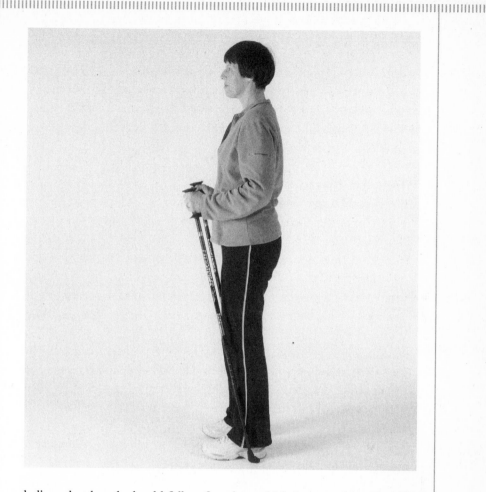

believe that length should follow function, which is easy with adjustable poles. Fittrek recommends poles long enough for the forearms to be at a slight upward slope for Nordic Walkers whose energy is "full power, standard and fast." For regular on- or off-road walking, the forearms should be as close to parallel with the ground as possible, and with forearms sloping slightly downward for speed.

LEKI has developed a chart for setting their three-section adjustable poles to the proper height. The suggested height is what the company calls the pole's baseline setting. The middle section can then be fine-tuned for comfort or conditions—usually shortened slightly on a prolonged uphill or it can be lengthened for a downhill—or if that is in your comfort zone, it can be lengthened for more aggressive walking.

Where to Buy Nordic Walking Poles

Nordic Walking poles are available from several sources: from retail stores (either independent or chain stores), from online retailers or on-line directly from the makers or from instructors affiliated with a particular brand. These are factors to consider when deciding where to purchase Nordic Walking poles:

When You Buy at a Brick-at-Mortar Retail Store:

- Your purchase is instant. You don't have to wait for your poles to be shipped to you.
- You don't pay shipping charges, or decide whether to pay more for expedited service.
- You can try the poles to determine whether the grips and straps are comfortable for you, which is particularly important if you have sensitive or arthritic hands.
- You benefit from the expertise and advice from a salesperson who has been trained by pole companies on the benefits of various models offered by the particular brands the store carries.
- You can make sure that fixed-length poles are the right length for you.
- You can try before you buy if the retailer organizes an introductory group walk that includes the use of poles.
- You support your own community (or a resort community you are visiting) with retail jobs and sales tax.

When You Buy Online, Phone Order or Mail Order:

- You can buy Nordic Walking poles whether or not any retailers in your area are enlightened enough to carry them.
- You can shop at your convenience, 24/7, and won't use gas or spend time doing so.
- You can easily comparison shop, pricewise, and decide among various sources: dedicated online merchants, direct from manufacturers, the online segment of a retail business or through eBay or amazon.com.
- You can order telescoping (adjustable) poles without worrying about getting the correct size.

- An important caveat for online shopping is that buying an off-brand, especially one offered at a too-good-to-be-true price, might result in a poor-quality product that will not withstand much use. The pole shaft might bend or even break. The metal tip or rubber paw might wear out quickly. The pole grip might be of an inferior material. Such online purchases may not carry enforceable warranties.

When You Buy from an Instructor:
- You have had the opportunity to use that particular model or that particular brand from the very beginning. You might have become comfortable with the poles on which you learned because they are the only type you know, but you are comfortable with them, and that's important when you go out on your own.
- You can immediately begin practicing what you have learned, while enthusiasm is still high and you remember what you were just taught.
- The price will be favorable, because instructors typically buy poles at a dealer discount and frequently pass on some of the savings to participants in their classes.
- You are helping the instructor stay in business to keep introducing others to the activity you have surely come to love.

Some people go into a retail store, pump that sales staff for information, leave and order online from some other enterprise. That simply isn't right—and in addition to the ethically questionable practice, it could discourage the retailer from continuing to cater to stock poles when he really isn't catering to a Nordic Walking clientele.

Pole Brands

Many long-time manufacturers of ski and trekking poles now also make Nordic Walking poles. As of 2009, the following brands of Nordic Walking poles are on the market. I give only some of the key characteristics of each at this writing. As you read this rundown, bear in mind that product modifications might be made to the cosmetics or features of any pole line, and models may be added or dropped, so what you see down the road could be very different from the list here. In any event, more information is available from retailers and on each manufacturer's Web site. When you are researching poles, check the availability of replacement policies for a specific period, perhaps one year from date of purchase, especially if you are buying an inexpensive set of poles. A bargain is no bargain if a pole bends or breaks after a few months' use, so look for a company that stands behind its products. A few brands carry lifetime warranties, which is something also to be considered if you intend to be a frequent and energetic Nordic Walker.

In addition to the brands below, of course, new ones will most likely appear, and lines may change as Nordic Walking finds its footing on the fitness firmament. Also, you may occasionally see custom pole brands on the trail. For instance, Exel makes three models of poles for Peter Schlickenreider, a German cross-country ski champion who is also a high-profile Nordic Walking promoter who has filmed a popular instructional series on one the Bavarian television network. For complete contact information for the brands below, see the "Resources" section on page 159.

What's in a Name?

What we call "poles," Brits and their Commonwealth cousins (except for Canadians, who speak more like us south-of-the-border types) refer to as "sticks." This is a close transliteration of the German word, *Stöcke*. The French call them *batons*. The linguistically gifted Scandinavians tend to use English words when they are not speaking to fellow Finns, Swedes, Norwegians or Danes.

BOOMYAH
The Tone 'n Trek pole is an easy-to-use, well-priced pole adjustable aluminum model introduced in 2008. Its signature color is a distinctive orange, appearing on every pole, but it is more than just a different face. This pole, initially available in just one model but several color combinations, introduces unique features to Nordic Walking that were not previously available from any other manufacturer. A soft, cushiony grip is topped

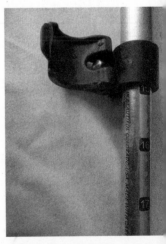

Boomyah's E-Z Flip Lock system for height adjustme

with a push-button quick-release mechanism for the strap. The strap itself is intuitive and has an easy Velcro closure and no buckles. Adjusting the pole is also easy, whether loosening or tightening the strap or lengthening or shortening the shaft. The Velcro accommodates different-size hands, gloved or not, and pole length is adjusted without twisting the two parts of the shaft. Instead, the user flips open a simple locking mechanism, slides the two parts of the shaft to the desired length and closes the lock. Pole length markers on the shaft make it simple to adjust both poles to exactly the same length. The rubber traction foot is larger than most, and it is somewhat keyhole-shaped to fit correctly into the somewhat key-shaped base of the pole so that it is impossible to position it at the wrong angle. Other features include sand/snow basket and reflective safety strip for night visibility. You're probably wondering what Boomyah means. It's shorthand for "Boomer—Young at Heart," expected to be the biggest growth area for Nordic Walking.

Boomyah International LLC, www.boomyah.com

EXEL

Exel Oy (*oy* being Finnish for industry) was established in Finland in 1960 and is a supplier of such diverse products as industrial tubing, building frameworks, lattice masts for airport lighting, tool handles, telescopes— and Nordic Walking poles. In fact, this is the pole brand that initially put Nordic Walking on the European map and has made great strides in doing so in North America as well. Exel quite accurately calls itself "The Original Nordic Walker." In 2008, Karhu Sports, another Finnish company and a major presence in cross-country skiing equipment, purchased Exel and revamped its product mix. The 2009 line of Exel Nordic Walking poles was pared down to five one-piece models, down from 13 models two years earlier. They range from the high-end Nordic Walker Extreme to the Active for the occasional Nordic Walker. In between are the Sport, the Trainer and the Stride. Shafts are different grades of carbon-fiber. Grips are either cork or one of several synthetic formations, and most of the straps are of various ComFit designs. A rubber paw fits over each tip for use on asphalt or pavement. Exel poles are made in 5-centimeter increments from 100 to 125 centimenters. Exel also sells angled tips and snowshoe baskets. The old Exel sold grips, straps and baskets separately for replacement of individual components, but it is unclear whether the new one also does.

Exel USA, www.nordicwalker.com

EXERSTRIDER

Wisconsin-based Tom Rutlin, who established Exerstrider in 1988, is committed to strapless poles. ERGO/SC grips are ergonomically shaped to provide unrestricted comfort and eliminate straps that he believes some users find complicated or uncomfortable. Exerstrider poles are made of aluminum alloy with hardened tungsten tips and trademarked Cushiongrip caps that fit over them. The poles come in a range of sizes for people from 4 feet, 11 inches tall to 6 feet, 8 inches tall. In addition to this classic one-piece pole is the newer OS2 Fitness Trekker adjustable pole that can be fitted to Nordic Walkers between 4 feet, 2 inches tall and 6 feet, 2 inches tall. For a slight price premium, a version suitable for individuals up to 6-feet, 8-inches tall is available. Perhaps the two extra-long poles should be called Exerstrider's NBA series. An Exerstrider product, introduced in 2007, is the Activator Medisport Edition, the first pole that specifically addresses the needs of older Nordic Walkers with serious mobility problems, arthritis and the like. This innovative adjustable-length pole utilizes the same kind of snap button/hole-length adjustment mechanism commonly used on canes and walkers—and therefore familiar to people who have been using walking aids, physical therapists and caregivers. It also features Exerstrider's strapless ergonomic grips. There are two rubber paw options: the boot-shaped Cushiongrip rubber tips and an optional bell-shaped balance tip for those with balance problems.

Exerstrider Products, Inc., www.exerstrider.com

FISCHER

This major Austrian maker of Alpine and Nordic skis and poles, tennis racquets and hockey gear for a time made eight models of Nordic Walking poles for the European market. They were never imported into the US, and in 2007, according to Fischer Sports USA, the company stopped selling them in Europe when the sport's growth curve there flattened and the market softened. However, they are still occasionally seen in Europe.

Fischer Ski, www.fischer-ski.com/en/nordic_walking

FITTREK

In 2000, Florida-based fitness expert Dan Barrett founded Fittrek. He began manufacturing walking poles under its own brand name 5 years later. There are currently 4 adjustable models. Distinct features are the Quick-Switch mix-and-match strap and tip systems and the Quick-Adjust two-section poles that can be adjusted with a couple of twists. The shafts, which carry a lifetime warranty against breakage, are made of extruded, seamless, aircraft grade-aluminum. Three interchangeable straps suit activity, and even hand size and comfort: Cross Trainer Straps, medium wide and well cushioned "for trails and heavy use;" wider Velocity Straps "for lightweight speed and comfort;" and Hands-Free Straps that most closely resemble ski-pole straps, "for those Nordic Walkers that prefer unrestricted use of their hands." Similarly, the Quick-Switch tip system offers three options to accommodate different surfaces and uses: Pro Tips for energetic Nordic Walking, Traction Tread Tips for wet surfaces, and the Low-Profile Basket that slips on for sand or even snowshoeing. Each pair of poles comes with all three straps and all three tips.

An illustrated instructional manual also comes with every set of poles, and Fittrek sells accessories and value-added packages to accommodate Nordic Walkers who are seeking an accelerated workout that incorporates strength training. The Power Belt is a fully padded strap-on belt with resistance cables that clip onto the poles. Patented reels called Power Packs provide two levels of resistance over the full range of the arm swing while walking. Think of it as a cross between Nordic Walking and Bowflex-style strength training. This optional add-on includes the Power Packs a pair of Nordic Walking poles, Traction Tread Tips, an instructional manual, a 90-day fitness plan and a "quick sheet" designed to help learn Fittrek's technique quickly and easily.

Fittrek, www.fittrek.com

GABEL

See Stride, below.

GYMSTICK

Like the pioneering Exel, Gymstick is a Finnish company. It came onto the fitness scene with three innovative products. In addition to poles for Nordic Walking, the others involve a single pole with resistance bands for gym/home and water/pool use. The one-piece fiberglass walking poles come in 90- to 130-cm lengths with plastic foam grips, ergonomically designed straps, metal tips, air cell paws and built-in resistance bands or coils built that can easily be pulled out from the shafts to add a strength-conditioning component to a Nordic Walk and make it into an interval workout. Two levels of resistance training bands can be selected.

Gymstick, www.gymstick.net

IWALK2

Iwalk2 are very affordable, adjustable aluminum-alloy poles imported by a sister enterprise to the Canadian Nordic Walking Association. Two models are offered. The Fitness Expert comes with a synthetic EVA/cork grip, a beefy rubber paw and a clip to hold a pair together. The Walking Expert has an EVA grip, to which the straps are affixed via a small wedge that holds them in place. An optional release strap, small and large baskets (the latter for snowshoeing), a clip to hold poles together, and a couple accessories such as waist pack and water bottle are also available.

Iwalk2, c/o CNWA/Timberdoodle Outdoors,
www.timberdoodleoutdoors.com or http://cnwa.info/

JOY

This innovative Swiss pole, which is not currently imported into the U.S., features a click-in/click-out strap and a patented, easy-to-use swivel tip adjustment, called tip2pad. This ingenious system that changes the metal tip to the natural rubber pad and vice versa. The metal tip retracts into and emerges from the rubber paw with a turn of a locking mechanism. The shaft is made of heavy-duty but lightweight carbon-fiber, and the wide straps come in S, M and L to fit comfortably, regardless of hand size or whether the user is wearing gloves for winter Nordic Walking. These one-piece poles are offered in 90- to 140-centimeter lengths.

Balanced GmbH, www.balanced.ch (Web site currently in German only)

KEENFIT

These affordable adjustable poles, nicknamed "Walkeen" poles, are delivered with three pairs of rubber paws and baskets, a value-added bonus. Made of aluminum alloy with a cork grip and a quiet, one-twist locking device, they come in two-piece (recommended for everyday use) or three-piece (recommended for traveling) versions that are amazingly accommodating for Nordic Walkers from 4 feet to 6 feet, 5 inches tall. They are offered in a rainbow of colors. They come with two pairs of feet or paws. One set of paws has a flat, angled bottom and is meant for asphalt or pavement. The other pair with rounded bottoms is intended for trails with compacted surfaces such as gravel. Without either set of paws, the carbide steel tips alone are for use on some hiking trails or on icy trails. Also included is a basket for use on sand or for snowshoeing.

Keenfit, www.keenfit.com

KEYTZ

These poles are manufactured especially to be sold on amazon.com. Click on "About Us" on the Keytz Web site, and up comes the notice that they are an Amazon Services Product via Brandswest, which also distributes LEKI poles and a variety of other health and fitness products. Made of carbon and aluminum, Keytz adjustable poles come in black, white or pink. They come with rubber paws for pavement that may also be purchased separately. Their most significant attributes seem to be that they are inexpensive and are delivered to the buyer's door.

Keytz Poles, http://keytz.com; Brandswest, www.brandswest.com

KOMPERDELL

This leading Austrian pole company manufactures a series of ultra-lightweight poles featuring high-quality carbon, bamboo or combination shafts; cork or foam grips and high-quality straps made with specially processed leather. The straps have a reputation for being comfortable and are designed to keep pressure off the wrist. Seven models are currently available. The Featherlight series comprises fixed-length poles, the Vario series poles are adjustable and the Nordic Blading model is designed with a longer shaft and other modifications specifically for in-line skating with poles. Komperdell poles are currently imported to North America directly by REI in the U.S. and MEC Sports in Canada.

Komperdell, www.komperdell.com

LEKI

This important German pole maker, founded in 1954 and known for its ski and especially trekking poles, offers more than a dozen Nordic Walking models in North America (and even more in Europe) and has been instrumental in promoting Nordic Walking in the United Sates. LEKI makes adjustable and fixed-length and also a travel model that fits into a suitcase. LEKI started its Nordic Walking pole line with models that were "slightly modified versions" of its trekking poles.

Now, poles are specifically made for Nordic Walking with expedition-weight aluminum, carbon-fiber or combination shafts, narrow-profile "cross-country"-style grips with adjustable/releasable trigger straps—making LEKI the most important Nordic Walking pole brand with such convenience. The Instructor series, which can be considered LEKI's bread-and-butter poles, are two-piece poles made of aluminum and carbon. Other features include carbide tips, removable rubber paws and baskets. LEKI says that the Super Lock System used on its adjustable poles provides "optimum locking" with less tightening torque than most adjustable poles. The company reports that it has been tested by TUV, a leading international testing, evaluation and certification organization, as "the strongest system in the world, with 360 degree reverse turn security and 140kg holding force."

The Speed Pacer Vario models are adjustable within a 10-centimeter range, meaning that, for example, a 125-centimeter pole can be customized within the 120- to 130-centimeter range, with an adjustment mechanism in the pole grip rather than in the shaft as with the conventional twist/lock type. The aluminum shaft of the Vario XS, a kids' model, adjusts from 80 to 110 centimeters. Instructor and Supreme poles have a twist/lock system. The Traveller series' all-carbon shafts collapse to just 26 inches. Other LEKI features include the brand's Shark Grip handle, excellent wrist support, carbide tips, several styles of removable rubber caps and optional baskets. One cap model resembles an auto tire, with deep treads and a curved shape that some people find more ergonomic. Another, which resembles a studded snow tire, has blunt metal studs embedded into the bottom to provide traction on ice or extremely hard-packed snow. Two types of adjustable/releasable trigger straps combine superior wrist support with the convenience of click-in/click-out release.

LEKIUSA, www.leki.com

NORDIXX

The Nordixx Global Traveler is a lightweight, three-section adjustable pole that fits into most suitcases (even in today's carry-on era) and are therefore especially suitable for travel—just as the name indicates. The aluminum-shaft poles are adjustable from 31 to 83 inches to fit walkers from four feet, nine inches to six feet, five inches in height. The straps click in and out of the ergonomic EVA-coated handles. Removable rubber paws for on-road use slip over tungsten or carbon-steel off-road pole tips.

Nordixx, www.nordixx.com

POWERWALKER

These Walker's Warehouse low-cost adjustable poles are promoted via amazon.com and can be used with fitness celeb Denise Austin's Powerbelt Walking System resistance device.

www.walkerswarehouse.com

POLEABOUT

This Australian company burst onto the Nordic Walking world with tremendous credentials. Signed onto the team are such luminaries as Marko Kantaneva, who was instrumental in launching Nordic Walking in Europe and who continues to promote it internationally; Michael "Walking Wizard" Gates, who is messianic about walking with poles for health and fitness; Meredythe Pembroke, 50-plus grandmother who became the first woman to pole-walk for 24 hours in the Finnish endurance challenge in 2006; Jay Gates, a multi-sport enthusiast well-known in Australia, who counts walking with poles as one of his many favorite activities; and Peter Oliver, who came back from a heart attack to complete 24 hours of pole walking at Tweeds, Australia, in 2007.

PoleAbout makes several models of adjustable poles in two sizes that are tagged "general" and "small." They are offered with four handle options (economical plastic, soft or hard rubber and natural cork), Velcro straps and three shaft options (carbon-fiber composite, composite fiberglass and aluminum alloy). The easy-use feature of the round rubber paw simply involves lining up the nose of the paw with the nose of the basket and pushing it onto the tip. PoleAbout products are available in Australia, the U.K. and several European countries, but not currently in North America.

PoleAbout, www.poleabout.com

SKIWALKING

SkiWalking's moderately priced, user-friendly one-piece VIP poles feature comfortable patented straps, durable carbide tips for snow, ice, beach and unpaved trails and removable natural rubber fitness paws for pavement and even indoor use. Customers who buy poles from SkiWalking's Web site are not asked what length they want, but what their height is. The company then matches the correct pole length to each walker's height, with a perfect-fit guarantee that the poles will be shipped in the proper size for the customer. In addition to its own brand, SkiWalking also is a leading seller of Swix poles (see below). In fact, Swix makes SkiWalking poles as well. Pete Edwards, who promotes the use of one-piece poles over adjustables, not only developed these poles, but also the American Nordic Walking System progression.

Skiwalking, www.skiwalking.com

STRIDE

Stride poles are made by Gabel, a well-known Italian pole manufacturer established in 1956. Several models, from recreational to professional, are available. Shafts are aircraft-grade aluminum or composite containing 50 percent carbon-fiber. As style-conscious as an Italian company is expected to be, it presents its walking pole with shafts in a half dozen colors and striking color combinations. Pole grips are either cork or synthetic, and click-on straps are available.

Gabel USA, www.gabel-poles.com

SWIX

Swix Sport is headquartered in Lillehammer, Norway, site of the 1994 Winter Olympics. This highly regarded cross-country ski pole and ski wax company, which was founded in 1947, makes both fixed-length and adjustable Nordic Walking poles. The carbon-fiber shafts are topped with cork grips and patented straps, but most of all, this brand became known for a patented, lightweight Twist & Go dual tip that easily changes, with a quick twist, from tungsten (metal) to rubber, or vice versa. The company also offers apparel for fall and winter workouts.

Swix Sport USA, Inc., www.swixsport.com

A Word About "House-Brand" Poles

As Nordic Walking grows in popularity, you will find more house-brand or private-label poles in a variety of outlets, both online and at brick-and-mortar retailers. Most of these poles, (which are manufactured in the Far East, mostly in China or Taiwan) are sturdy, and all are moderately priced, but they often do not have the technical refinements or comfort features found on more expensive, name-brand models. And in some cases, you truly get what you pay for and might find that off-brand poles are more likely to bend or break. If price is your only consideration, they are the way to go. If not, shop around. Quality and durability do cost money, but dedicated Nordic Walkers find worthwhile the additional price for a known brand.

The bottom line is that with Nordic Walking poles and good shoes (see next chapter), you're set to become a Nordic Walker. The next step, literally and figuratively, is to get out and do it.

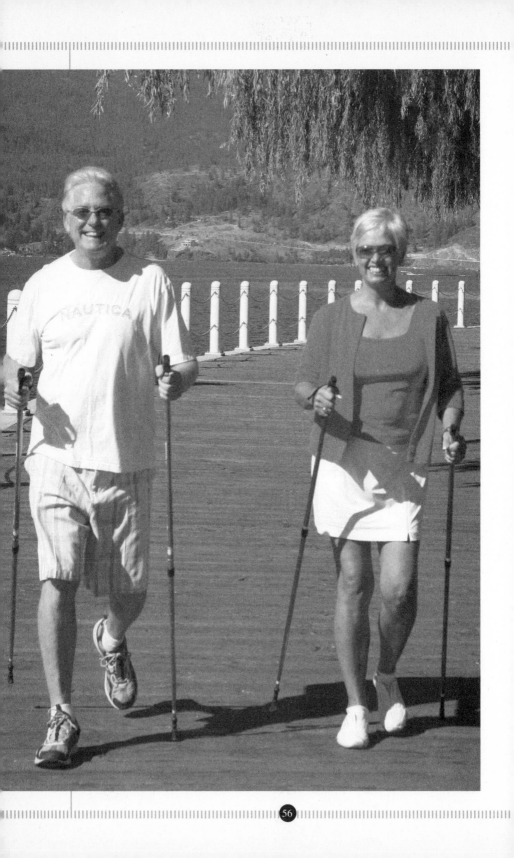

Gearing Up:
Shoes for
Nordic Walking

The single most important quality for any shoes you buy—in fact, the only really important thing—is proper fit. Beyond that basic requirement, the two next most important qualities for Nordic Walking footwear are sturdiness and comfort—or perhaps, comfort and sturdiness. If you find a perfect match between your feet and one particularly well-fitting sports shoe brand and size, those are the shoes for you, regardless of the activity for which they were designed. Not surprisingly, Nordic Walking shoes are best suited for Nordic Walking. They are widely available in Europe but still less so in North America, where manufacturers and importers want heavier participation and a promise of rapid growth before they distribute and market such a specialized product. Many sporting goods and shoe retailers are similarly conservative about carrying products for an activity that does not yet have a proven market. Because Nordic Walking is a relatively new sport here, it might therefore be difficult to find a pair in the first place, let alone a pair that fits you well. In that likely case, try walking shoes. If you are an urban Nordic Walker and plan to walk mainly on pavement or asphalt where you won't need a beefy tread, walking shoes will probably work well for you,

If you can't find any suitable walking shoes, try trail running shoes, which are stiff laterally and therefore supportive. By contrast, regular running shoes meant for pavement are designed to provide cushioning rather than support. The differences between walking and running footwear reflect the biomechanical differences between these two activities. Quality running shoes are particularly well cushioned along the sole, because of the strong heel strike and the relentless pounding that runners' feet, legs and entire bodies undergo with every stride on pavement. Because walking in general and Nordic Walking in particular are low-impact activities, the shoes should be stronger at the heel to facilitate a continuous heel-to-toe movement with each step. Shoes made specifically for Nordic Walking are stiffer in the heel section and more flexible in the forefoot section than regular walking shoes and certainly more so than running shoes. Of course, they are also supportive underfoot and well cushioned to provide a measure of shock absorption. Further, they often also mitigate either pronation (rolling the foot and ankle inward) or supination (rolling them outward). Shoes should have removable insoles so that you can add orthotic inserts to mitigate those common conditions and help your feet achieve and maintain a neutral position. (See Chapter 4, "Toys and Togs").

If you intend to do all your Nordic Walking in and around town, on paved paths, sidewalks or lightly trafficked roadways, and perhaps on relatively flat dirt and gravel paths, walking shoes with fairly smooth soles will do. But if you are going to go trail walking on steeper, rockier or uneven terrain, look for footwear with a decent tread. Many dedicated Nordic Walkers prefer to wear light day-hikers on such trails, though do try to find these low-cut hikers with the most flexible possible soles—and don't even think about wearing ankle-high hiking boots for Nordic Walking. If you live in a hot area, look for shoes with ventilated uppers to help perspiration evaporate. If you live in a wet, rainy area, you may want shoes lined with Gore-Tex, Dryworks or some other waterproof membrane to keep your feet dry.

Some people swear by shoes with negative heels (that is, a heel section that is lower than the midfoot and forefoot) or shoes with rocker soles (higher in the midfoot section than at the heel or forefoot). Negative-heel designs have been around for a long time. Earth Energetic has been making this style for decades, while SpringBoost incorporates the concept in its more recent Nordic Walking models with one of its interchangeable insole designs. MBT, which calls itself the "anti-shoe," (see page 64) claims that the rocker sole "transforms flat, hard, artificial surfaces into natural, uneven ground. Much like walking in sand, the unique action…challenges the core, strengthening muscles to be more active. This reactive, more supportive muscle action creates good posture and increases shock absorption for all the joints, significantly reducing muscular-skeletal compression." The "walking on sand" analogy might seem like a bit of a stretch, until you realize that some people who do their Nordic Walking on hard, wet sand near the waterline actually do so barefoot.

Assuming, however, that you will be wearing shoes, you need to make sure that you buy the correct size (including width). You can use orthotics to tweak shoes that do not fit your feet perfectly. These footbeds are not, to paraphrase an old car commercial, your grandfather's arch supports. For more information, see Chapter 4, "Toys and Togs". The information contained in the "Footwear Brands" section below was researched in 2007. Models often change from year to year or season to season. Some changes are simply cosmetic (new colors or color combinations) or in name (a new model name given to an existing design), while others are fundamental to the fit and function of the shoes. A good and knowledgeable shoe salesperson will know the difference.

Shoe Shopping Tips

- To find footwear with proper fit and appropriate functionality, go to a specialty sports shoe retailer or runners' store that carries a number of brands and also has a sales staff with expertise in fitting footwear for active sports. These merchants are a better bet than a discount shoe store or big box retailer—and much better than mail order.
- If you have a pair of walking shoes or running shoes that you have used for walking, take them along. An expert can tell a lot about your feet, your stance and your walking style from the way you have broken in your footwear.
- Shop for shoes in the mid- to late afternoon, bringing with you the socks you prefer to wear with athletic footwear.
- Brand loyalty accounts for a lot in people's buying decisions, but be open-minded and try others as well. You may go back to your favorite, or you might surprise yourself and find some that you like even better.
- If you are interested in such unconventional designs as negative-heel or rocker-sole models, you need to put previous shoe-shopping

experience aside when you try them on. It is important to isolate the issue of correct fit from the fact that your foot position in the shoe (and therefore your steps) will be unfamiliar. In other words, try not to misinterpret the "weird" sensation of standing or walking in them with poor fit.

- A good salesperson will make sure that your feet are not squashed by the shoes, that there is about a half-inch between the end of your longest toe and the front of the shoe, that you have sufficient width in the forefoot, and that the heel fits snugly.
- Select shoes with removable insoles in case you need or want orthotics to fine-tune the fit and just about customize the shoes for your own feet.
- When you buy shoes, wear them at home for a few hours so that if you need to exchange them, they will be clean.

Footwear Brands

Theoretically, it is possible to go Nordic Walking in any comfortable footwear from Tevas to Crocs, especially on fairly flat paved or packed-dirt surfaces, but in practice, specialized footwear is safer, more comfortable and more effective in maximizing the benefits of fitness-walking with poles. If this were a European book, there would be quite a number of brands listed, because more companies there make or distribute footwear just for Nordic Walking. And if this book were coming out a very few years down the road, there would most likely also be more brands offering Nordic Walking shoes. However, this is North America, where specialized shoes remain few. Most Nordic Walkers will therefore be satisfied with "regular" walking shoes for walking on pavement and smooth, packed trails. Even when specific shoes are sold in various countries, they often carry different model names in Europe and in North America, so use the information below just as a guideline to what is available out there—at least at this writing.

While many conventional walking shoes sport relatively flat, flexible soles, a contrarian concept imported from Europe is gaining adherents in North America. As noted earlier, several brands of shoes feature some sort of negative heel design, which mimics the motion of a bare foot walking in soft sand. This might be via a "rocker" sole that is thicker under the instep than at the toe and heel. This curved shape is designed to propel the foot straight through the heel-to-toe motion of each step. Fans of such footwear—currently made by Chung Shi and MBT—credit the shoes with pain relief, improved posture, a more natural gait, and reduction of stress on the knee and hip joints. Somewhat similar in concept are negative-heel shoes like Earth Energetic and to a degree, SpringBoost with one of its interchangeable insoles. Like Nordic Walking itself, this category of footwear helps stimulate unused and underused muscles, thereby increasing core strength and specifically improving below-the-waist muscle tone. Some advocates also claim that rocker-sole design also makes the legs shapelier and combats cellulite—whether used with or without poles. Manufacturers' specific product groups and models within each group change from year to year. Established companies might introduce specific Nordic Walking models or begin addressing the needs of Nordic Walkers in the general walking shoe collections. Styling and color choices are up to you; they don't affect performance, which is what is addressed here.

ADIDAS

This sports footwear and active sportswear giant currently offers six men's and eight women's models that it says are suitable for walking. Some are light trail shoes; others are cross-trainers. Noteworthy for anyone who is Nordic Walking often in wet conditions is the Mali, with a "water-grip" outsole.

Adidas US, www.shopadidas.com and www.adidas.com/us/

ASICS

Asics is a Japanese athletic shoe manufacturer founded in 1949 as Onitsuka Co., Ltd. The name Asics was adopted in 1977. Its own Research Institute of Sports Science has made it a leader in footwear and apparel innovation. The GEL-Yeti WR was Asics' first shoe designed for Nordic Walking, but since Nordic Walking didn't take off as quickly as the company would have liked, Asics has "repositioned" it as a regular walking shoe. It is still suitable for the fitness activity for which it was designed. The shoe's rugged outsole offers traction, Asics' trademarked GEL Cushioning System provides shock-absorption and the water-resistant, heavy-mesh upper is lightweight yet sturdy. Asics' European divisions distribute up to six models of specific Nordic Walking shoes, so don't be surprised to see more styles available and positioned as Nordic Walking shoes when the market grows in North America.

Asics America, www.asicsamerica.com

BROOKS

This high-tech British shoe company currently includes in its line the Cascadia model, sized for men and women and meant specifically for Nordic Walking. Its trademarked Dual Pivot Posts are designed to accommodate the destabilizing effect of trail irregularities. HydroFlow cushioning units are designed to dampen shock and rebound on every stride, and the line also includes other performance features. It is currently not widely available in North America.

Brooks, www.brooksrunning.co.uk

CHUNG SHI

This distinctive shoe with the Chinese name is actually from Germany. The name was inspired by the traditionally uneven walking surfaces in rural Asia that assured healthy body alignment. To add to this internationalism, Foot Solutions, which at this writing has 200 retail specialty shoe stores, is the exclusive U.S. distributor of Chung Shi shoes. Adherents consider the shoe with the rocker sole to be effective in promoting a natural rolling motion when walking (or jogging) and a natural upright stance, improving posture, absorbing road shock, strengthening core muscles, and improving circulation in the legs and feet. It "meets the guidelines for medical products and is a Class 1 Medical Device," according to company literature. The Chung Shi shoe comes in two versions, the Comfort Step with a 15-degree-angle sole and the Balance Step, a more aggressive 20-degree-angle version. Chung Shi footwear is designed for a soft heel strike and a natural forward-rolling action that is biomechanically sound, and a midsole "air bag" serves as an arch support. Fans say that it improves circulation, relieves back and joint problems and even offers a reflexology-style foot massage while walking.

Chung Shi, http://chungshiusa.com

EARTH ENERGETIC

This environmentally and socially conscious company has been around since the early 1970s, producing performance fitness and walking shoes for men and women. They are best known for their patented Kalsø Negative Heel Technology, which promotes good posture and enhances the stride. A Danish yoga teacher and student named Anne Kalsø developed this concept, in which the heel is lower than the forefoot and toes, which was inspired by the way locals walked in the sand when she studied at a yoga monastery in Santos, Brazil. Now, the full line of patented footwear includes walking shoes whose full heel-to-toe layer of Gelron 2000 minimizes impact to the heel, leg and lower back. Other features include removable sock liner, carbon-fiber shank for support, and leather and mesh uppers.

Earth Energetic, www.earthfootwear.com

EASY SPIRIT

As one of the first companies to address the specific needs of walkers rather than runners and other active sports participants, Easy Spirit has a reputation for making shoes that combine comfort and performance for walking and light running. Hard-to-fit feet are also an Easy Spirit specialty. Among the women's models that appear in the walking-shoe line at this writing are the Pacifico, Powerplay, Speedrate, Sightsee and Hittheroad, all cushioned and designed for fast-paced walking. Romy and Headsup are suitable for more casual walkers, and Jumper has been designed for intermediate walkers. Wintrtrail is a sturdy shoe with a deep tread for good traction. Easy Spirit's Perfect Fit program accommodates a range of foot sizes and shapes. However, at this writing, the status of the line's walking-shoe collection was uncertain. The Jones Apparel Group, a conglomerate of fashion brands, owns the brand and could change the direction and positioning.

Easy Spirit, www.easyspirit.com

INOV-8

Inov-8's 13 models of trail-running and trail-racing shoes, including some for women, have found favor with Nordic Walkers who like the stability, lightweight ruggedness, low cut and aggressive soles of this kind of footwear. All are suited for trail walking, even under daunting conditions. The British company's top seller is the Roclite 285.

Revel Sports, www.revelsports.com

LOWA

This venerable German company appears to recommend all of its active sports shoes for Nordic Walking. Nine men's models and eight women's models currently comprise the Outdoor Fitness/Trail Running category. The Mira XLR LO Lady, which Lowa calls an "ultra-lightweight hybrid," seems well-suited for Nordic Walking as well as day hiking. Features include a Cordura "collar" for comfort, Gore-Tex XCR lining, polyurethane midsole and liner, and New Bite rubber sole for grip and stability.

Lowa, www.lowaboots.com

MBT

Karl Müller, a Swiss engineer who had suffered from back pain, was so inspired by the Masai people's natural, comfortable barefoot walk that he designed shoes to mimic that physiology. The line's initials stand for Masai Barefoot Technology. MBT shoes are designed to stimulate the body to balance itself and promote natural muscle function that replicates "walking barefoot on springy moss or a sandy beach." The implication is promotion of a comfortable, natural stride. When Müller used his own design, he reported that his back pain disappeared. MBT footwear utilizes a patented rocker sole, the Masai Sensor to create the "natural instability" of the barefoot walk, a fixed polyurethane midsole and pivot to activate the body's stabilizing muscles, a firm shank to create the foot's natural rolling motion and an insole for comfort. MBT shoes are made in men's and women's sizes, with the two-tone style Lami, a retro-chic model styled and sized for women.

MBT, www.swissmasaius.com

MEPHISTO

Manufactured in France, Mephisto's Rush for women and Match for men are pricy, high-quality, handcrafted walking shoes made of top-grade, water-repellent natural and nubuck leathers. Other features in the Rush include an anatomic arch support, Air-Jet for midsole air circulation and two-point air-bag shock absorber at the heel and under the metatarsal arch to secure protection of spine and joints. Match boasts the Air-Relax System for extreme breathability and durability and the Air-Jet circulation system throughout the midsole. A dynamic two-point Air-Bag System is incorporated into the lightweight latex foam sole. Both men's and women's models include anatomic insoles and padding on top to reduce pressure points from the speed lacing system.

Mephisto, www.mephisto.com

MERRELL

Merrell's line changed radically for 2009 with six women's models and three for men recommended for walking. The women's Siren Sync is especially well cushioned for comfort, while the beefed-up Siren Sport Gore-Tex XCR is also completely waterproof. The ultralight Paragon is a running shoe with minimal weight. Pantheon is a dedicated men's walking shoe. Radius is waterproof and has aggressive lug sole. Riot in men's and women's sizes is designed for city streets. Merrell also makes a collection of comfortable outdoor action garments.

Merrell, www.merrell.com

MIZUNO

Mizuno got its start in 1906 and with growing sales of such Western sports gear as baseballs, quickly expanded to made-to-order athletic wear and beyond. By 1912, it supplied shoes to the Japanese team at the first Olympics in which the country competed. Runners value Mizuno because models include the Neutral model for feet with normal pronation, the Support model for moderate pronation and the Control model for severe pronation. The opulently cushioned Wave Rider series is recommended for walking.

Mizuno, www.mizunousa.com

NEW BALANCE

New Balance began making arch supports in the early 1900s and in the '70s expanded to produce athletic footwear. It has since grown into a leading supplier of fitness products.

The New Balance 1091 is a multi-sport shoe that adapts well to Nordic Walking. Introduced in 2007, it is lightweight (12 ounces) and designed with a Dryworks membrane waterproof upper to keep feet dry. To accommodate the Nordic Walking heel-to-toe foot motion, the shoe's patented Abzorb heel and forefoot offer shock absorption. Other patented features include the TS2 Transitional Support System to help control pronation and to provide a smooth transition through the gait cycle, and the N-Lock provides mid-foot support and a snug feel. For trail walking, 1091's gusseted tongue is designed to keep pebbles and other debris out of the shoe. Additionally, New Balance produces two categories of traditional walking shoes for men and women: Athletic Walking Shoes for both competitive and casual walkers (12 models each for men and women) and Country Walkers (5 models for women, 4 for men) for off-road recreation, plus one model for serious race-walking. These shoes are known for their wide range of sizes (5 to 20) and widths (AA to 6E). The New Balance 759's forgiving mesh upper stretches to accommodate wide feet and even bunions. The 858 is built with extra ankle stability. New Balance's patented features, offered on the appropriate models, include the Rollbar for stability through the stride and Abzorb SBS in the heel for enhanced shock absorption.

New Balance, www.newbalance.com

THE NORTH FACE

The North Face got its start as a modest sporting goods store catering to San Francisco's climbing community in the freewheeling 1960s. Some two decades later, it began manufacturing packs and later clothing, all designed for rugged outdoor use. To underscore its commitment and seriousness, the company's slogan became, "Never Stop Exploring." After more than four decades, The North Face delivers an extensive line of performance apparel, equipment and footwear. The company's trail running shoes for men and women are especially suitable for Nordic Walkers who prefer rough trails to manicured urban paths. The shoes are built to be both supportive and cushiony, including an EVA midsole on some models for extra cushioning that makes them especially suitable for rocky trails. The Rucky Chucky has a harness that wraps around the foot and a zigzag Snake Plate underfoot that further enhances both medial and lateral support.

The North Face, www.thenorthface.com

REEBOK

Reebok traces its history back to J.W. Foster & Sons, its "ancestor company" founded in England in the 1890s, and literally and figuratively began hitting its stride at the 1924 Olympics—the Games whose runners were celebrated in the film, *Chariots of Fire.* The current Reebok, although now part of the Adidas family of companies, retains its distinct brand identity that projects a hot, with-it image despite its long history. The Reebok name now appears on highly functional footwear and apparel for active sports. The women's Premier Verona

KVS is the heir to the Premier GTX, a dedicated Nordic Walking shoe. Features include the Kinetic Fit System with comfort, support and flexibility where they are needed. This design also includes walker-friendly forefoot grooves to enhance flexibility, rugged outsoles for traction and removable sockliners to accommodate orthotics. EasyTone is a walking shoe with built-in "balance pods" to enhance toning similarly to the negative-heel and rocker-sole concept. Smoothfit SelectRide's hidden-seam construction is comfortable for walkers and runners with sensitive feet. Several of the men's running shoes, notably the Premier models, are also suitable for walking.

Reebok International, Ltd., www.reebok.com

RYKÄ

Rykä was founded by a woman and remains true to women's needs. Sheri Poe founded the company in 1987 to create the kind of well-fitting active footwear that she herself wanted. Now privately owned by American Sporting Goods Corporation, Rykä continues the mandate of making performance fitness products for women. High-tech active footwear is designed to a woman's last need with a narrow heel and a wider, more forgiving forefoot. The two-decade-old company currently makes half-dozen mid-price walking shoes from casual, about-town models to true performance models. Ranging from the most aggressive to the most casual, they are Moira, Country Muse, Muse Walk, MC Walk, SportWalker Inspiration and Pace Walk.

Rykä, www.ryka.com

SALOMON

Salomon's Walker Fit, sized for men and women, is a robust, supportive shoe specifically designed for Nordic Walking, featuring a lightweight, quick-drying upper, Contragrip soles for both durability and grip, a protective synthetic toe cap and asymmetrical speed lacing. The Walker Comp is similar but softer. The Walker Softshell in women's and children's sizes is softer still and has fewer high-tech-sports features but still works for some Nordic Walkers, especially those who use paved routes and find closed shoes uncomfortable. The Gore-Tex-lined XA Comp 2 XCR is a rugged shoe suitable for foul-weather Nordic Walking.

Salomon Outdoor, www.salomonoutdoor.com

SAUCONY

While Saucony does not currently make a specific Nordic Walking shoe, it does produce highly technical walking shoes and also running shoes for men and women. The Grid Motion 6 is a sleek men's and women's shoe with full-grain leather in the forefoot, support at the instep and midsole and, to provide comfort for some hard-to-fit feet, stretch zones at the first and fifth metatarsals (those long bones leading to the big and little toes).

Saucony has several features (including patented ones) that are incorporated into its walking footwear. Among them is a web of woven synthetic filaments that provides cushioning and stability, and centers the heel on impact of every step. HRC (High Rebound Compound) is an EVA/rubber compound that cushions the metatarsal area. The Midfoot Support Bridge is a rigid material in the shank of the midsole to keep the foot neutral during the step-gait cycle. The company currently markets three models of walking shoe: the ProGrid Stabil LE 4, the Grid Omniwalker and the Grid Motion 6, all sized for men and women. The women's Grid Omni Walker comes in narrow, medium and wide widths; the men's in medium and wide. The men's and women's ProGrid Stabile LE 4 is offered in medium, wide and extra-wide. The women's Grid Motion 6 is offered in narrow, medium and wide and the men's in wide only.

Saucony, Inc. www.saucony.com

SPIRA

Embedded in the soles of Spira shoes are one large mechanical spring under the heel and/or two smaller ones under the forefoot—respectively single-spring, dual-spring and tri-spring configurations—known as recoil footwear. This trademarked WaveSpring system is touted as returning energy back to the runner or walker with every step. The company calls it "recycling" energy and says that it combines this energy return with cushioning. Several dual-spring models of men's and women's walking shoes are part of the Spira line, but some Nordic Walking authorities believe that the shock absorption provided by springs mitigates the power push-off that is necessary for upper-body toning.

Spira, www.spirafootwear.com

SPRINGBOOST

This Swiss-made performance shoe is a relatively kid new on the Nordic Walking block, that burst on the stage with models of specially designed shoes. Dorsiflexion is the distinctive feature of the technically advanced B-Walk Nordic Walk model. If you're wondering what "dorsiflexion" is, according to SpringBoost, it's "a position whereby the heel is lower than the forefoot." In other words, a negative-heel design. SpringBoost shoes are sold with two sets of interchangeable insoles, enabling users to get used to the sensation with an insole at zero degrees dorsiflexion and then to kick it up with a 2-degree dorsiflexion insole.

SpringBoost, www.springboost.com

TIMBERLAND

Timberland traces its roots to Boston in 1918 and the Timberland name to 1977. It has been a major player in the sports and casual footwear market ever since. Timberland's Iduion Nordic Walking Shoe didn't make a major impact in the North American market, so the company went after Nordic Walkers in Europe, where the line has been more successful. In North America, the shoes were well received, but retail merchants were reluctant to devote space to them in their stores. "We didn't have a ton of broad success," according to Timberland's Janet Brennan. "The shoes were great. So unfortunately this is one of those programs that only lasted a season." Four models are currently on the market, distributed primarily in Europe but also available through some online merchants.

The Timberland Company, www.timberland.com

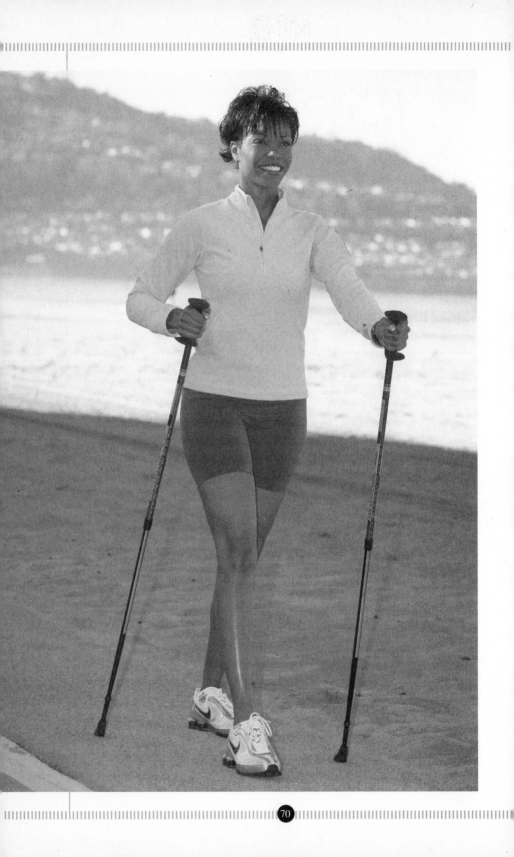

Toys
and
Togs

No one heads out for a Nordic Walk with nothing but poles, shoes, and perhaps a few fig leaves. Some people dress down, grab their poles and head out the door, relishing the simplicity and freedom of the activity. Others like to have the latest in active wear and add all manner of accessories, from special clothing accessories to fancy electronic devices—pedometers, heart rate monitors and such that keep track of the length and duration of the walk. Other people like to listen to music. Still others need to find a way to handle both Nordic Walking poles and a dog's leash. But when it comes right down to it, poles, shoes, socks and something more concealing than those fig leaves are the gotta-haves that no Nordic Walker can be without. The rest are optional products to enhance the Nordic Walking experience—products that might be called wanna-haves. This chapter explores some of the options in clothing and gadgetry that fall into both the gotta-have and wanna-have classifications.. There are also a few items, such as orthotics, that fall into the very-good-for-most-people-to-have category. If you have been a hiker, runner, walker or exerciser, you probably already some of these items. Otherwise, start with the basics, and add on as needed.

GOTTA-HAVE ACCESSORIES

- Socks
- Custom orthotics or other footbeds (for many, even most, people)
- Sunscreen
- Hat (for sunny or rainy situations)
- Gloves (for cold or rainy situations, or simply to protect the hands)
- Underfoot traction devices (if you regularly walk on hard-packed snow or ice)
- Hydration pack or water bottle holder (for all but the shortest walk)

WANNA-HAVE ACCESSORIES

- Small daypack or waist pack
- Tieless shoelaces
- Personal identification item
- Pedometer (this verges on the gotta-have, and you'll probably soon find yourself moving it there)
- Heart-rate monitor
- Holder for iPod or other audio-entertainment device
- Dog-leash system

Brand names are given here not as endorsements but as examples of products—some familiar, others less so—that are on the market at this writing. Sporting goods stores, running stores, retail shops at fitness centers and gyms, sporting-goods catalogs and online merchants carry some or all of these items.

FOR THE FEET

Shoes are the most obvious products you will wear on your feet. Socks, replacement laces, orthotics and a few other optional accessories are below-the-ankle items that some Nordic Walkers can't live without.

SOCK IT TO YOUR FEET

Well-fitting, totally functional footwear demands good socks. More important, the health and comfort of your feet demand good socks. What are the definitions of "good"?

- Good socks are the right size for you and fit your feet snugly to prevent blisters.
- Good socks are appropriate for the season.
- Whether of a synthetic or natural material, good socks wick moisture from your feet.
- Good socks are formed with flat seams for comfort and also to protect against blisters.
- Especially if you are susceptible to athlete's foot or other fungal conditions, good socks are antibacterial or antimicrobial.
- Especially of you are prone to blisters, good socks can be constructed of two thin layers rather than a single thicker layer.
- Good socks are lightly padded to provide additional conditioning in order to alleviate fatigue on long walks.
- And it should go without saying that good socks are not worn thin and don't have holes in them.

Sox Appeal

In this era of renewed appreciation for natural materials, it is tempting to pick up a six-pack of cotton sports socks and call it good. Perhaps surprisingly, cotton is the least suitable fiber for long walks because it retains moisture in the summer or in a year-round hot climate, and it does not keep feet warm in the winter. Whatever the season or the climate, cotton can stretch and shrink and therefore is unlikely to retain its shape as well as synthetics or blends. Polyester is the generic umbrella term for numerous brand-name synthetics—perhaps blended with such synthetic fibers such as nylon, polyacrylic, polypropylene, Lycra or other elastic and even Teflon, as well as wool, a natural fiber.

A few companies make specific walking socks. Others make running socks, fitness socks or general sports socks that are suitable for Nordic Walking. Many Nordic Walkers who live in extremely rainy areas have taken to wearing waterproof socks made for bicycling and off-trail/ endurance running. Whatever their primary purpose, socks come in various heights and styles (and even colors and designs). These of course are more a matter of personal taste than function, but function should always come first.

For summer wear, when your feet are likely to perspire, CoolMax is arguably the best-known fiber for socks in the running and walking communities because of is moisture-wicking properties. CoolMax, one of many brands developed by Invista, a leading supplier of integrated fibers and polymers, is also woven into fabric for active sportswear as well as socks. The large spaces between the filaments of the fibers are like little ventilators, drawing moisture from the feet and promoting breatheability to keep them cool. Among the sport sock brands using fast-drying CoolMax are Asics, Assos, DeFeet, Fox River, New Balance, Rohner, Save Our Soles (SOSS), Thorlo, Wigwam and WrightSocks. If you do extensive off-trail walking where gravel and grit can enter the shoetops, another model to consider is Revel Sports' anatomically designed Debris Sock CoolMax, a single piece that combines the gaiter and sock, to keep dirt out.

The polar opposite of CoolMax is ThermaStat, a DuPont material that is suitable for winter walking socks. This hollow-core fiber, which traps insulating air and lends itself to double-layer construction, is composed of very fine filaments designed to retain warmth to keep your feet toasty. This fiber also wicks moisture which is important on long, cold walks, because cold, wet feet are uncomfortable at best and can be frost-nipped or even frostbitten at worst. ThermaStat is designed to heat up rapidly and to retain warmth as well. Among the sock brands using ThermaStat are Assos and Running Room. ThermaStat is also used for skiing and snowboarding socks, meaning that they are particularly warm and can also be used for Nordic Walking in a very cold climate. But you'll have to try them with your walking shoes to determine whether they would work for you—or even consider two pairs of walking shoes, one for warm weather and one for cold.

Teko's tekoPOLY line is made of recycled polyester—both post-consumer and post-industrial material—for its performance sport socks that offer excellent moisture transfer, have a soft hand, dry quickly and are durable. The Quarter Cut model is good for Nordic Walking.

While cotton can be a problematic natural material in a walking sock, wool is a natural material that does what you would expect it to. That is, it not only keeps feet warm when it is dry but also retains its insulating properties when wet—hardly trivial for Nordic Walking under cold, damp conditions. SmartWool, the leading brand of wool sport socks, makes machine-washable socks. Teko's tekoMERINO socks—the Quarter Thin, Light Hiking Thin or Quarter Cut models being particularly appropriate for Nordic Walking—are made of wool from sheep ranches that are committed to sustainable agricultural practices, and the EcoWash Merino versions are also machine-washable. Rohner, a Swiss specialty sock manufacturer known for high quality, makes the "original super-light" sock with a patented non-slip tube and wool-blend weave for fitness-walking.

Rohner makes socks for fitness and wellness that are suitable for some people's particular needs. Wellness socks from Rohner include several models with additional under-instep support, and its patented SeaCell Active models are made with SeaCell Active, a cellulose fiber that sounds like a vitamin supplement or natural food additive. It includes "active algae ingredients" and a bit of silver in the materials mix. Rohner claims that the addition of "trace elements, carbohydrates, amino acids and vitamins" are released by ski contact, while the silver enhances both anti-bacterial and wicking qualities. The Anatomic Trail and Silver Runner models are among those that come in left and right socks, like gloves or shoes, for maximum comfort.

And—drum roll—Rohner even makes a sock especially for Nordic Walking. "Reinforced areas at the toe and heel have positioned exactly on the zones that take the strain when walking," the company says, adding, "The elastomer in the instep area assures good grip in the shoes. CoolMax FX works antibacterial and odor-inhibiting. CoolMax and high-quality wool in the sole provide optimum conditions for feet and maximum comfort." Leave it to the Swiss; a few bumps in the translation of their catalogue copy notwithstanding, but this is a sock made with quality ingredients and real forethought for functionality specifically for Nordic Walking.

YakTrax's merino wool socks for men and women feature a trademarked Thinvent mesh top for breathability, a deep heel pocket to minimize foot movement and friction, and patented slip-resistant ribs to reduce shear. The instep area is shaped for secure fit and arch support, the hand-looped toe seam is comfortable during the end of each stride and the wool's inherent cushioning without bulk provides a comfort bonus for long walks.

Whether you buy socks based on functionality, price or on your conscience—or a combination—keep in mind that a comfortable, wrinkle-free fit is the most important characteristic.

GOTTA-HAVE SHOE ACCESSORY

Orthotics occupy their own special niche between what every Nordic Walker must have, accessory-wise, and what some Nordic Walkers want. For most people who spend a lot of time on their feet, some sort of underfoot support is required just to get through the day, and when the exercise of choice is walking, the benefit of good orthotics is maximized. A custom pair can make a lot of difference for endurance, comfort, foot health and even knee and hip health.

Making the Shoe Fit

Few people are fortunate enough to have perfect feet that fit perfectly into those perfect shoes. Custom orthotics, footbeds or at the very least, simple off-the-shelf arch supports compensate for pronation and can alleviate foot discomfort, foot pain or even real foot problems. They are inserted into the shoe, normally under the insole (which is a good reason to buy shoes with removable rather than glued-down insoles) to correct abnormal or irregular walking patterns and make fitness-walking, regular walking and even standing more comfortable. Stores that sell running or walking shoes, as well as podiatrists, can make orthotics. You will be fitted with whatever brand is preferred there.

Rigid orthotics are made of carbon-fiber or some kind of plastic that is custom-molded to your own feet. This relatively thin footbed is designed to stabilize the joints for more efficient and comfortable function. It can extend either from the toe to the ball of the foot for walking or all the way to the heel for therapeutic purposes. A pair of orthotics can last for years and can be moved from one pair of shoes to another. Remember that full-foot orthotics do not allow the foot to flex through the walking motion.

Soft orthotics are thicker and more cushiony underfoot to absorb shock, improve balance and relieve pressure from any uncomfortable or potentially sore spots on the sole of the foot. Made of soft, compressible materials, soft orthotics can either be molded by your feet as you walk or custom formed over plaster impressions of your feet. They usually extend from the heel past the ball of the foot to the toes. Unlike rigid orthotics, the soft variety does need to be replaced periodically.

Semirigid orthotics are favored for sports because they are designed mainly to provide balance and guide the foot through the proper motion while walking or participating in other sports for efficiency and even injury prevention. They are made of soft materials that are reinforced with more rigid ones.

Integrated Footwear System

Sock maker ThorLo in 2006 introduced its Exercise Walking System and has gradually eased it into the marketplace. It might be a one-shot wonder that never takes hold beyond this one company—or it might be an indication of things to come. While not specifically designed for Nordic Walking, the system addresses the needs of walkers with hard-to-fit feet or anyone who tends to experience discomfort with new shoes or when walking. It comprises a well-fitting, cushioning sock, a footbed designed to be both supportive and energizing and a lightweight shoe that reportedly requires no break-in. When people buy outdoor footwear, they tend to buy the shoe first, then perhaps pick up some socks and maybe even stick an old pair of orthotics into them. With this system—more than a decade in the making—the three main footwear components are designed and made to work together to provide both comfort and performance. The integrated approach comprises an exercise-specific sock, a footbed meant to go with the sock and the shoe, and the lightweight shoe itself that is available in various sizes and widths for men and women. The Exercise Walking System is most suitable for use on pavement rather than on unpaved trails.

WANNA-HAVE SHOE ACCESSORIES

While big corporations employ scientists, researchers and marketing experts to develop, produce and distribute big products, ingenious tinkerers and small entrepreneurs are in basement workshops and garages, busily identifying specific problems or annoyances, and developing modest products to solve them. The ones here are not specific to Nordic Walking, but are useful for it.

Lock Laces and Tyless Laces are clever and inexpensive devices to solve the small but annoying problem of auto-untying shoelaces. With Nordic Walking poles in hand (except with brands such as LEKI, Joy or Boomyah poles that have releasable straps), each stop is just a bit more involved than simply propping a foot on a curb or rock and retying the wayward lace because you have to remove your pole straps. These two products therefore have significant appeal to Nordic Walkers who prefer not to stop. Both are elastic replacement laces with a disk or button to hold them in place and maintain the desired fit on the foot without loosening the lace. When you are finished walking, unlock the gizmo to slip the shoes off. When you're ready to go next time, just slip your feet back in and tighten the lace-holder up again.

In the safety department, identification accessories that don't interfere with Nordic Walking are invaluable in the unlikely case of an emergency. If you're walking with a group or at least one other companion, a personal ID probably won't be necessary. However, if "something" happens when you're out on your own, wouldn't you want emergency personnel to know who you are and whom to call? Road ID's line of stainless steel "people tags" are laser-engraved with name, address, emergency contact information or medical alert (epilepsy, insulin-dependency, etc.). Models are available for the wrist, ankle and even shoelace. The Shoe ID is a simple tag that is attached to the lace of one shoe via a small Velcro strap, while the Shoe ID Pouch version also accommodates a credit card, key and a bit of mad money.

SKIP THE SLIP

Nordic Walking is genuinely a year-round activity, even in northerly climates where packed snow and ice are winter constants. The best investment you can make is a pair of traction devices that fit under the soles of your shoes or boots. Traction aids prevent slipping and twisting something or even falling and getting hurt. Even if you feel fairly sure-footed, you will walk less tentatively and get more benefit from each Nordic Walk if you are really confident on a slick or uncertain surface. Of the several brands on the market, most utilize cleats and all offer models for men and women.

STABILicers are made in Maine, a state where active outdoors folk have been innovators in developing gear for winter. Tubbs, America's oldest snowshoe maker, started in Maine. More recently, 32North, the company that makes STABILicers, is even located on a street called Arctic Circle. STABILicers' robust, all-purpose Foot Traction Cleats are abrasion-resistant, self-cleaning Vibram soles with embedded hardened-steel cleats that dig into hard snow and ice. STABILicers

Sport and Lite models are detuned versions designed for energetic walking and running with a natural stride. The company likens its STABILicer Sport Ice Grippers to studded snow tires for the feet. They fit over footwear with thermoplastic elastomer (TPE) caps that stretch over the heel and toe. Case-hardened steel cleats to bite into the snow, with replacement cleats are also available. The STABILicers OverShoe adds extra insulation on really frigid days.

Two other traction devices use criss-crossed springs or chains. Instead of cleats, lightweight YakTrax traction devices rely on tightly coiled springs of thermal plastic or steel that slip over the sole and crisscross under it. The coils' sharp edges bite into the slippery surface. YakTrax are rated to −41 degrees Fahrenheit. Kahtoola's MICROSpikes are heavy-duty traction devices for rugged snow and ice conditions—not for a little layer of ice on a smooth sidewalk or roadway. You slip your foot into what looks like a flexible rubber spat, and cinch it down. The underfoot traction component consists of a sturdy criss-crossed chain and 10 aggressive spikes. MICROSpikes come in sizes ranging from youth to large men's shoe sizes.

REFLECTING ON NIGHT SAFETY

If you walk at night, particularly along roadways, a little reflectiveness goes a long way to alert drivers to your presence. Many running shoes and some running apparel has small built-in panels of Scotchlite or other reflective material. Fittrek builds some reflectivity into its poles for safety when walking after dark, and Boomyah supplies reflective stickers that walkers put onto their own poles. Scotchlite reflective materials are available in small kits available in hardware stores. You can apply the material to just about anything. Also, Reflectively Yours, a mail-order outfit, distributes various do-it-yourself reflective materials that can be sewn on, ironed on, Velcroed on or stuck onto poles, garments and accessories. The firm's Runners Kit can also be used for Nordic Walking.

THE PARCH-PROOF NORDIC WALKER

Staying hydrated, which is modern sportspeak for drinking enough water, is critical for comfort and health—and an important component for weight loss or weight maintenance as well. Physiologists tell us that 60 to 70 percent of the composition of the human body, including the muscles, is water. We take it in by drinking, and we eliminate it through urination, respiration and perspiration. Nordic Walking and other exercise causes us to produce more heat. The body's response is to perspire in order to cool down and regulate temperature, which in turn requires drinking water to maintain that equilibrium between intake and output for comfort and health. Like any exercise, Nordic Walking makes the body to heat up and causes water loss (even in cold weather), and that lost fluid must be replaced during exercise. With poles in each hand, carrying a water bottle is obviously impossible.

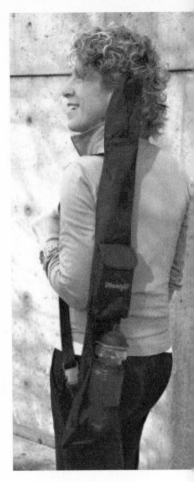

To remain hydrated no matter how long the walk, you need to take a water supply with you. Some walkers like lumbar or hip packs that hold one or two water bottle holders, plus a zippered pocket for carrying extra clothing, spare socks, wallet, keys, energy bars or other snacks, sunscreen and other necessities. For Nordic Walking, look for a model that you can adjust to fit you comfortably without banging against you with every step and that also is designed so that it does not interfere with your arm swing or your poles.

Hydration packs resemble small daypacks, with shoulder straps that leave your hands free for your poles. Inside the pack is a plastic bladder that usually holds between 1.5 to 3 liters of water. A long flexible tube with a bite valve makes drinking easy so no hands are needed during a walk. Many hydration packs also feature pockets, pouches and/or elastic cords so that you can carry the small items mentioned above and perhaps also extra clothing. Look for narrow shapes that won't interfere with your arm and shoulder motion, and of course, be sure that the straps can be adjusted for comfort. Several manufacturers make women-specific models designed for a better fit to the female form. CamelBak launched the hydration pack revolution. Other brands include Arc'teryx, DaKine, Deuter, Gregory, Kelty, The North Face, MSR and Platypus.

WATER OR WHAT ELSE?

The first rule of hydration is simply: don't wait until you are thirsty to drink. Thirst is a sign of the onset of mild dehydration; so drink before you start on a walk, and unless it is a very short one, continue drinking throughout. Water is the number-one liquid for staying hydrated. Under normal circumstances (meaning a moderate-length walk or a longer moderately paced one), water is really all you need. If you are walking hard on a hot day, perspiring heavily and breathing hard, you could be taking in as much as one quart of water per hour. Tap water, filtered or purified water and bottled water, including fancy designer brands and vitamin water, have the same effect on hydration. In other words, any kind of water does the same hydration job, though for comfort, you will want to stick to still, rather than sparkling, water before you go out.

There are options if you just can't abide a lot of water. One popular choice is tea that has no caffeine and no sugar, honey or other sweetener. Europeans, in fact, are fond of herb teas when exercising. Real fruit juice, not fruit-flavored drinks or fruit cocktails, is a good choice. Many people especially like to drink juice before or after a walk because it tastes so good.

Gatorade, which came on the market in 1966, was the first specially formulated sports drink. Sports drinks are formulated with about the same proportions of electrolytes—including potassium and sodium, sugar and perhaps some of the same nutrients as are found in the human body. Many serious athletes have come to depend on replenishing, refreshing sports drinks, and Nordic Walkers who go on particularly long, high-intensity training walks might find them beneficial too.

Unless you are working out at a high level, these products will give you calories you probably don't want and will replace electrolytes that don't need replacing. However, if you are really cranking for more than an hour or two, especially on a hot day, a sports drink can provide a boost. Gatorade, the first big brand of sports drink, is still around. The original is now simply called G and a low-calorie version is called G2. Its ever-evolving product line includes formulations designed for consumption from early morning to post-workout. Other sports drinks now on the market include All Sport, Accelerade, Clif Shot Electrolyte Replacement Drink, GU Sports GU2O, Gleukos Sports Fuel, Lucozade, POWERade and PowerBar Endurance. If you are Nordic Walking in Asia, know that the curiously named beverage called Pocari Sweat is a sports drink. CamelBak Elixir and Nuun Hydration Tablets are tablets that dissolve in water to turn it into an electrolyte-replacing sports drink, while Tang Sport is a quick-dissolving powder packaged in single-portion tubes that is designed for the same effect. It's not quite as miraculous as turning water into wine, but when you're lagging during a long walk on a hot day, you'll think it is.

Many experts caution people to avoid so-called energy drinks (as opposed to sports drinks), which are high in sugar, calories and caffeine. Caffeine is a diuretic, so caffeinated teas and coffee are also poor choices before and during exercise. Carbonated soft drinks, whether caffeinated or not, are also not suitable before a Nordic Walk.

Rehydrating after a walk is important too. Health-conscious purists drink more water, fruit juice or perhaps decaffeinated iced tea. In any case, avoid caffeinated drinks for a while after your walk. But for many people, especially Europeans who traditionally tap into the social and communal aspects of outdoor activities, this is the time to enjoy a beer. Drinking isn't the only way to rehydrate after a Nordic Walk. You can also slice a thick slab of watermelon. The flesh is 92 percent water and it's a delicious treat on a hot day. Furthermore, if you are concerned about nutrients, know that it also contains as much lycopene as four tomatoes—significant because lycopene is said to boost the skin's natural burn-protecting SPF, which in turn is important when Nordic Walking.

FOR THE NORDIC WALKING
GEEK IN YOU

If you are Nordic Walking for serious athletic training or for weight management, or if you have physician-mandated exercise parameters, a heart rate monitor and/or a pedometer falls into the gotta-have category. If you are a geek and a gearhead, they are wanna-have items that enable you to track your Nordic Walking workouts just for the fun of it. The descriptions below are overviews of what each item is, what it does and why it enhances your Nordic Walking.

Pedometer

What an odometer is to your car, a pedometer is to your Nordic Walking routine—an instrument that measures distance traveled—and often more. To simplify greatly, pedometers operate by measuring body motion. As you walk, your steps cause an abrupt change in motion, which in turn triggers the instrument's mechanism and registers on the display. In most models, a click of a button shifts from counting steps to measuring the distance you've walked—and multi-function models also have the ability to convert your steps into distance, separately display the number of aerobic steps that you have taken and perhaps even calculate walking speed. Today's pedometers may also include speedometers, stopwatches, calorie estimators, heart rate readers and more. They can track these statistics cumulatively, and many can interface with your PC. At the end of the day, or after several days, you can upload the information from the pedometer's memory to your computer via a cable that plugs into the USB port.

Some companies have gotten really creative in what they put into their pedometers. Sportline, for instance, makes one model that talks to you and another that you can talk to. The former has a robotic voice that announces your steps or distance, or alerts you when you have reached a preset goal of the day. The latter has a little built-in recorder so you can make audio grocery lists, business memos or add items to your to-do list that occur to you during your walk. You will, of course, have to release the grip on your poles while recording, but you'll be glad when you're through that you didn't lose any good ideas while you were out. The company also offers pedometers with a flashing safety light for nighttime walks or built-in FM radio.

Bells and whistles aside, at its most fundamental, a pedometer must merely count the number of steps you have taken since it was reset. An easy-to-read digital display and a practical design that makes it difficult to accidentally push reset or other buttons are features even of inexpensive but well-thought-out pedometers. Simple models are reset manually. More sophisticated ones reset automatically every day—or sometimes at whatever interval you establish.

You must calibrate your new pedometer to your stride length in order to display distance accurately. Before you begin using it, measure the length of your step or stride when you walk with poles. The easiest way to do this is by extending a carpenter's measuring tape on a sidewalk or down a long hallway. Starting with the toe of your front foot at one end of the tape, take 10 comfortable steps at your normal pace using poles. At your tenth step, see where the toe of the front foot on the tape. Divide by ten to get your stride or step length. Then, adjust your pedometer accordingly. The instructions will explain how. Pedometers are normally affixed to a belt or waistband with a main clip and often a small secondary clip on a little safety leash so that you don't dislodge the device accidentally and drop it. At least one brand, Highgear, makes a pedometer that is worn on the wrist. Some pedometers include instructions on precisely where to position them for the most accurate reading or distance; others are more forgiving. The step count should be very close to the number of steps you actually walked. At the end of the day, that's what matters toward your fitness, health or weight goal.

The simplest pedometers count steps. Period. Others also keep track of miles and/or kilometers, number of aerobic steps, calories burned, cumulative steps and other data. The Nike + iPod Sport Kit is more than even a complex pedometer alone. A wireless sensor designed to fit into Nike+ footwear transmits data to your iPod nano, which then either displays the data or "talks" to you via your music mix. Many brands are on the market, with astonishingly low prices for the most pared-down models. Among the brands that you will find in sporting-goods stores, running stores, online and elsewhere are Acumen, Accusplit, Bodytronics, DashPak, Fitbug, FitSense, Freestyle, Garmin, Highgear, Kenz, NB Monitors, New Fitness, New-Lifestyles, Nike, Omron, Oregon Scientific, Polar, Reebok, SportBrain, Sport4Life, Sportline, Timex, Total Fitness, Walk4Life and Yamax.

HOW FAR IS FAR ENOUGH?

When the topic of walking for wellness comes up, it's not miles or even speed that matters but number of steps. People have different stride lengths, depending on height, leg length and sometimes how flexible and active they are. Conventional wisdom is that an adult should take at least 10,000 steps a day at least 6 days a week to improve fitness or maintain good health. When you think of the increased benefit you get from walking with poles, it is clear that Nordic Walking gives you more bang for each walking buck. When you start a walking program, put on your pedometer first thing in the morning and wear it all day. You may find that you are walking several thousand steps just in your normal routine even if you have not been on any fitness program. Of course, to benefit your cardiovascular system and burn more calories, you need to make an effort to include a substantial number of aerobic steps—and that is where the Nordic Walking bonus kicks in. There is no hard and fast rule about this increase in activity. It depends on your starting point.

If you have really been sedentary, you can establish 5,000 steps a day as your first-level goal. If you have been sort of active, try for 7,500 steps a day at the beginning. If you're fairly active already, make 10,000 steps your initial daily goal. Depending on your stride length, that's roughly 5 miles. Some experts believe that a reasonable guideline for moving from sedentary to active is to increase walking by 10 to 15 percent in time or distance for each day and also for the total number of walks per week. Within 4 weeks or so, a healthy adult who started with a 5,000-step goal should be able to walk 10,000 steps most days of the week. No matter where you started, remember your pole—and use them. Once you have reached that 10,000-step goal, consider what's next. If weight loss is your goal, try to add 2,000 to 3,000 steps every day to that basic 10,000. If you want to enhance your aerobic fitness, make sure that at least 3,000 of those are fast Nordic Walking steps. Some pedometers actually count both total steps and aerobic steps to help you keep track of your level of activity.

Remember to put on your pedometer first thing in the morning. When you begin Nordic Walking, make a note of how many steps you took before you head out with your poles, and check the number of steps again at the end of your walk. As your fitness and stamina improve, try to increase both your Nordic Walking steps and your daily-life steps with such oft-repeated fitness tips as finding a more distant parking space from work or store, walking children to school, taking the dog out for a longer walk and taking a stroll during your lunch hour to increase the number of steps you take in a day. Keep a daily log of the total number and the Nordic Walking number. The greater both numbers, the better you'll feel.

Heart Rate Monitor

The old-fashioned way to measure your pulse is to put a finger or two on your wrist or neck, find an artery and count for 10 seconds. Multiply by 6 to calculate beats per minute, and you've got it. But times change, and some experts now caution against pressing your fingers against the artery in your neck so as not to impede any blood flow to brain. And, of course, in the fitness realm, the old-fashioned word "pulse" has now been replaced with the phrase "heart rate." In most non-athletes and non-medical thinkers, they are, for all practical purposes, the same thing. Now, as a further departure from tradition, there are electronic devices to continuously measure and monitor heart rate, especially when working out—and as a bonus, you don't have to stop walking to determine how you are doing. Overall health and cardiovascular endurance are improved by increasing those heartbeats through aerobic exercise.

You might wonder why checking your heart rate while you walk matters. The resting heart rate (RHR) is your heart's number of beats per minute while you are sitting or lying still. You want your heart and lungs to work harder—but not too hard, especially when you begin your Nordic Walking program. According to the American Heart Association, proper pacing during exercise is essential, explaining, "To receive the benefits of physical activity, it's important not to tire too quickly. Pacing yourself is especially important if you've been inactive."

Of course, it is also important to check with your physician and/or work with a trained fitness professional before embarking on a Nordic Walking program, especially if you have been sedentary or fairly inactive, but by understanding this basic information, you can begin to understand why heart rate is so important. By paying attention to your target heart rate (THR), you can monitor your progress as you embark on and continue a Nordic Walking program. Some people find it motivational in and of itself to track progress from week to week. The THR, which you might see referred to as the aerobic training zone, describes the ideal number of times per minute that your heart should beat while Nordic Walking or participating in any other aerobic exercise for fitness and weight-loss benefits. The THR is related to age (see accompanying chart). When you are finished walking and are cooling down, your body is in what is called the recovery mode. The better cardiovascular shape you are in, the faster your heartbeat slows down. People who train aerobically by the book follow formulas for warming up, reaching and maintaining a target heart rate and cooling down during the recovery phase back to the resting heart rate. Some athletes increase the effectiveness of their aerobic workouts with

American Heart Association Heart Rate Table

Here is the American Heart Association's table for estimated target heart rates for different ages (find the one closest to yours), as well as a couple of other simple guidelines and basic cautions.

Age	THR Zone 50–85 %	Average MHR 100 %
20 years	100–170 beats per minute	200 beats per minute
25 years	98–166 beats per minute	195 beats per minute
30 years	95–162 beats per minute	190 beats per minute
35 years	93–157 beats per minute	185 beats per minute
40 years	90–153 beats per minute	180 beats per minute
45 years	88–149 beats per minute	175 beats per minute
50 years	85–145 beats per minute	170 beats per minute
55 years	83–140 beats per minute	165 beats per minute
60 years	80–136 beats per minute	160 beats per minute
65 years	78–132 beats per minute	155 beats per minute
70 years	75–128 beats per minute	150 beats per minute

The AHA cautions: A few high blood pressure medications lower the maximum heart rate and thus the target zone rate. If you're taking such medicine, ask your physician or health care provider whether you need to use a lower target heart rate.

The AHA gives the following advice to those starting an exercise program: Aim at the lowest part of your target zone (50 percent) during the first few weeks and gradually build up to the higher part of your target zone (75 percent). After 6 months or more of regular exercise, you may be able to exercise comfortably at up to 85 percent of your maximum heart rate. However, you don't have to exercise that hard to stay in shape.

Initials to Remember, Heartily

RHR = resting heart rate
HHR = healthy heart rate
MHR = maximum heart rate
THR = target heart rate

interval training, which, at its most basic, alternates short periods of all-out aerobic effort and a pullback to recover. But all this is beyond imagining for the many people who are attracted to Nordic Walking because of the wellness benefits just from getting out and walking with their poles a few times a week.

For anyone who wants to parse these numbers even farther (and if you're a Nordic Walking wonk, you may), these percentages can be broken down even more for specific starting points and goals. If you have been sedentary or have been rather inactive, aim for the lower end of the range until you become fitter and stronger. The 50 to 60 percent range is a comfortable range that is sometimes called the healthy heart rate (HHR) zone and is beneficial while minimizing the risk of overexertion. If you have been active, try to stay in the higher range of this zone. Kick it up a notch to 60 to 70 percent to burn the most fat. Higher percentages—70 to 85 percent—are considered the aerobic zone, which are fat-burning too but are beneficial in really strengthening your cardiovascular system. Remember that as your fitness level improves, you can remain in this aerobic zone for longer periods of time, which in turn maximizes the benefit of each Nordic Walk.

The old-fashioned way to determine your target heart rate uses arithmetic and depends on age and gender. First, subtract your age from 220 if you are a man or 226 if you are a woman. That is your maximum heart rate (MHR). Your target heart rate is as low as 50 percent and as high as 85 percent of your MHR—though most people who have been Nordic Walking for some time aim for 65 to 75 percent range for both fitness enhancement and fat burning.

Today, many active exercisers prefer to use a heart rate monitor. Functioning like a portable, personal electrocardiogram device, it registers your heartbeats and therefore makes it easier to monitor and keep a record of these numbers—much as a pedometer does for counting steps. The typical heart rate monitor consists of two parts: a wireless sensor strap, worn around your chest under your clothing, (or is built into some sports bras), and a display unit that you wear on your wrist. It looks much like a digital wristwatch and continuously displays your heart rate in beats per minute, plus all sorts of optional additional information—as with pedometers, depending on the technical sophistication and price. There are also heart rate monitors with sensor touch pads that read your pulse off your index finger, but most experts do find these less accurate than those with chest straps. PowerGlove makes a monitor that resembles a glove that only covers the heel of the hand, part of the palm, the thumb and the wrist, but that design would seem to interfere with the grip and strap of the Nordic Walking pole.

Among the other features that you might appeal to you, especially if you love electronic gadgetry, are a stopwatch mode that can tell you how long you have been walking; an alarm that enables you to set your THR and warn you when you are falling above or below your range; a calculator that figures elapsed time and time in or out of your THR range; a calculator that estimates calories burned, and a download feature that interfaces with your computer to record your heart rate stats. Combine this input with statistics collected by your pedometer, and you will have quite a detailed Nordic Walking training log. Or, you can do it the old-fashioned way and write your statistics in a logbook

Some brands of heart rate monitors that you will find in retail stores and online are Cardiosport, Nike, Polar, Sportline, Suunto and Timex. Not surprisingly, several of these companies also make pedometers. If you get into super-serious training and are also concerned with your oxygen usage, the HD Pulse Oximeter is a small, easy-to-use device that measures and displays pulse oxygen saturation (SpO_2) and pulse rate. Stick your finger into the oximeter, and see an instant readout of your numbers.

STRIKE UP THE BAND!

If you Nordic Walk with a group or a partner, conversation is probably all the entertainment you'll need. But if you are a solo Nordic Walker, a little music will go a long way to keeping you moving, diverted and therefore devoted. The thrill that runners, walkers and other exercisers felt when the Sony Walkman was introduced in 1979 was multiplied in 2001 when the iPod, MP3 and other personal media players came along. These devices have spawned an entire accessory industry of holders that make it easy to be physically active with your most motivational music coming through your earpieces.

To take the player along on your Nordic Walks, you need a compact, lightweight holder configured so that the wire and earpiece don't interfere with the poling motion. Here's a trio of very different iPod holders that are on the market at this writing:

- LimbGear's Go-Sleeve is a double-pocket Polartec armband that slides onto the arm and secures with a quick twist to serve as an all-purpose accessory that firmly holds a cell phone, keys, cash, ID, lip protector and personal little sound system. I-Sleeve is its single-pocket alter ego. *www.limbgear.com*
- SportWrap is a slimmed-down version of a holder that can be worn on the upper arm or forearm. Two adjustable Velcro straps secure the iPod nano or other player, no matter how aggressively you move. The little built-in cleat keeps any excess earphone cord out of the way. The pouch is water-resistant and allows full access to the controls—though it won't hold your poles for you while you tinker with the buttons. *www.xtrememac.com/cases/nano_2g/sportwrap/*
- Sugoi's Audio-T shirt has a little pocket on the sleeve for an iPod or MP3 player. The earpiece and wire feed from the pocket and through the shirt and loop round the collar. Made of performance fabrics called TechniFine Mesh and TechLite, the shirt features ventilating mesh inserts. *www.sugoi.com*

WHAT TO WEAR OUT THERE

"I'm going Nordic Walking, and I have nothing to wear!" This is, of course, an imaginary lament, because just about everyone already owns suitable clothing. All you really need is something comfortable to move in and appropriate for the weather wherever you are. Consider that runners and cross-training athletes are out rain or shine, heat or cold, and use their dedication as a model—and perhaps shop where they do for comfortable, functional clothing. The principle of layering is pretty simple. With garments of different materials and functions, you can adjust to changes in weather conditions during your walk, as well as compensate for your own body heat as you work out with your poles.

On benign spring and fall days, or in winter in the sunbelt, almost any loose-fitting, comfortable clothing that permits a range of motion will work. You pick it—shorts, tights, T-shirt, sweatshirt, knit top, tank top, Lycra workout wear, runner's singlet, sweatpants, yoga pants and so on. When it's very hot, very cold or very wet, the choice of clothing must take functionality, and not just comfort, into consideration.

As with socks (above), cotton can be problematic. A cotton T-shirt might be just perfect on a warm spring day, but cotton retains moisture from perspiration and does not dry easily or quickly. In the heat of summer, it soaks up perspiration and hangs on to it. As soon as you stop working out hard, you might feel sweaty and icky. In cold weather, cotton stays wet, feels clammy and cold and can make you feel chilly at the very least or become hypothermic at worst. When wet, cotton has no insulating value and can cause real chills if the temperature drops. Cotton jeans are not desirable either, both because of the cotton fiber's inherent flaws for outdoor activities and because the heavy seams can be uncomfortable or chafe. Some people prefer Lycra or other stretch tights. Others prefer loose-fitting running shorts, long pants or sweat pants. The choice is yours. Whether you walk in long or short pants, an elastic waist is non-restricting and comfortable in motion. Again, as with socks, you'll want to look to the world of synthetic fabrics for the best functionality in many situations. In warm or temperate yet dry climates, you can go Nordic Walking in street shorts, running shorts, tights, capri pants, sweat pants, yoga pants, workout wear, long- and short-sleeve T-shirts, sweatshirts—depending on your own taste, what other walkers in your area wear and what makes you the most comfortable. A treasured cotton T-shirt and a pair of shorts are usually just fine in, say, Phoenix or San Diego, but in colder, wetter, less-predictable places, you'll need to be prepared for the outdoors with more versatile clothing. In such circumstances, the secret is layering.

Active outdoor apparel has not been the same since Malden Mills introduced Polartec, the first important brand of nylon fleece or pile. Made in various thicknesses, it is now the insulation material of choice. Many brands of this highly functional, super practical, machine-washable, quick-drying material are cut and sewn into a seemingly endless variety of shirts, jackets, pullovers, vests, neck gaiters, pants, hats and gloves. Stretch fleece is an insulated material that competes with Lycra for use in activewear tights.

In wet places or during the rainy season, you'll want to add a rain jacket and perhaps even rain pants. In warm, rainy locales, a light shell made of ripstop nylon finished for water repellency or water-repellant polyester microfiber that can be stashed in a pocket or on your hydration pack will do. Same concept applies to windy areas or windy days. When it's cold, a polypropylene base layer and a fleece jacket are suitable. For cold and windy conditions, you'll want an insulating layer and a shell over that. And when it's wet and/or cold and/or windy, a higher-performance waterproof/breathable outer fabric is just the ticket. Gore-Tex, the first such breakthrough fabric, is still the standard by which all others are judged, and garments made of the company's Windstopper material are insulating, moisture transmitting and wind-resistant—a trifecta of outdoor comfort.

In 2007, Lands' End introduced the Sport Collection of clothing specifically for Nordic Walking, becoming the first activewear line to address the specific needs of men and women who walk with poles. This is a very big deal for Nordic Walking, because Lands' End is a very big company. Two fabrics are used in the bulk of the first Lands' End Nordic Walking collection. Both are the company's refinements and applications of materials found to be particularly well-suited to multi-season outdoor activity. The company is committed to producing outerwear to keep people moving and comfortable, even as temperatures drop. Garments are made from fabrics that boast such properties as stretch, anti-static, wicking/breathable, antimicrobial, water protection and high-SPF ratings all geared for for Nordic Walking performance, comfort and maintaining warmth without chilling.

Vests and long-sleeved jackets are made with ThermaCheck fleece that is treated with a process called Nano-Tex Resists Static to resist static electricity build-up to prevent bunching—not to be dismissed with an activity that potentially involves brushing fleece-clad arms against fleece-clad torso. Jackets, capris, pants and shorts are made of Active Knit, a stretch fabric that wards off moisture and also is anti-microbial to combat odor—also not to be minimized. A versatile water-repellent jacket, a quick-drying tee that also "manages" both moisture and odor and long-sleeve base-layer tops called Thermaskins round out Lands' End's inaugural Nordic Walking line. And some of the tops are equipped with a pocket for an MP3 player or other personal entertainment device.

Winter Clothing

For winter Nordic Walks, take your cue from cross-country skiers and snowshoers, who have different gear underfoot but have exactly the same clothing needs. What they wear, and what you should wear too, is:

Base or Inner Layer: Worn next to the skin, the fabric must be wicking to transport moisture away from your body. Polypropylene is the generic favorite. Cool-Max is a brand that you'll often see. Tops come in zip-front turtleneck, crew neck and V-neck designs. Except in the most extreme cold, most Nordic Walkers won't need polypro bottoms, but they are available. You'll find them anyplace that carries skiwear or winter climbing and mountaineering garments

Mid-Layer: Again, synthetics rule. Polyester fleece tops come in various thicknesses, styles and a rainbow of colors and are lightweight, compressible and insulating even when wet. When it's cool but not cold, and/or moist but not wet, you will often wear this as your outer layer.

Outer or Top Layer: This is your first line of defense against wind and rain, so a quality waterproof, breathable fabric is mandatory if you expect to be out in heavy weather. Because it is worn on top of other insulations, you don't need a lined or insulated outer garment but rather one that is protective against wetness and wind. A water-resistant shell is the very least you'll want. More likely, a waterproof, breathable garment—seam-sealed to prevent moisture from seeping in—that continues to transport wicked moisture away from your body and yet keeps rain out will assure comfort during your walk.

DO SWEAT THE SMALL STUFF

Don't literally sweat the small stuff—you'll likely be sweating enough on your walks—but figuratively keep these other accessories in the forefront of your thoughts on gotta-haves or wanna-haves to be more comfortable and safer.

- **Headgear:** Depending on where and when you walk, your wardrobe should include a brimmed hat to wear when the sun is strong and a warm one for winter. Vented baseball caps, mesh-crowned or vented hiking headwear (often with chinstrap to hold it on your head in case it gets windy), or visors are options for summer. Fleece or wool designs that pull down over your ears are suitable for winter walking. Some people prefer headbands. Variations include sweatbands for summer, and fleece or wool to protect your ears and forehead in winter.

- **Sunscreen and/or insect repellent:** Sunscreen of the appropriate SPF is a must, year-round, and products that protect against both UV-A and UV-B rays are now widely available. Many people, especially women, prefer a gentle product to use on the face and throat. For other exposed skin—including the back of the neck, décolletage, arms, hands and legs—select products specified for "sport" use are formulated not to dissolve from perspiration. If you live in a buggy region, you might think that you can walk faster than any mosquito or other insect can fly, but it is also easy to walk into them if they are in your path. An application of insect repellent will have them veering away from you. Some products act both as sunscreen and insect repellent.

- **Sunglasses:** Style is not as important as protection. Make sure that they are rated to filter ultra-violet rays, which can harm your eyes. In addition to sun protection, shades keep the wind and even grit out of your eyes.

- **Pack:** If you only go for a short walk close to home, sticking your keys in your pocket might suffice. Otherwise, you'll need someplace to put "stuff." In addition to carrying water—whether around your waist or on your back, and whether a hydration system or a belted water bottle holder—you might want a small pack for essentials such as keys, cell phone, small wallet or purse for a bit of money and identification, sunscreen, energy bars, tissues, extra clothing, whatever. Choices are packs that are belted around your waist or that slip over your shoulders. In any case, try them on while walking with poles make sure that the straps are comfortable and non-restrictive, and can be adjusted to fit you.

- **Gloves:** The extremities—toes and fingertips—are more vulnerable to the cold than any other body parts, even when the thermometer doesn't read extremely cold. For winter and even for cool spring and fall walks, warm lightweight gloves might also mean the difference between frigid fingertips and comfort. Various kinds of stretchy fabrics, including fleece, are available. Again, if you walk in the rain, make sure that those gloves are water repellent too. It might seem a tad extravagant, but if your fingers still get cold in winter, you can buy single-use chemical heat packs that you can slip into your gloves. Place them inside your gloves at the backs of your hands, where the blood vessels are close to the skin. However, since they are not supposed to be directly on the skin, you'll also need a thin glove liner. Some people like to wear lightweight gloves for Nordic Walking year-round to prevent the pole straps from chafing or irritating any part of the hands. You can try cross-country ski gloves for winter walks, but test the combination of your poles and the gloves before you go out for a long walk. Some just are incompatible because of competing straps, buckles or Velcro closures.

- **Sports bra:** Ladies, Nordic Walking is no activity for sexy, flimsy, lacy and/or underwire bras. It requires supportive designs meant for active women. You'll want wide straps, a wide back panel and a size that keeps you from jiggling but doesn't confine uncomfortably.

Doggone Clever Leash Systems

You don't have to make a choice between taking the dog for a walk or going Nordic Walking. In order for their canine companions to join them and yet have free hands for their poles, Nordic Walkers have often tried to rig up some way to attach the leash to their waists. Several innovative products on the market do that.

In addition to being a leash-and-collar combination, Sporn Products' Multi-Leash offers a built-in option for using it as a belt leash, tied around the waist. The nylon leash has reflective stitching (should you wish to Nordic Walk with your dog after dark), is adjustable from 4 to 7 feet, and is offered in 3/8-, 5/8- and 1-inch widths. To deal with an eager dog that likes to pull, the company's Non-Pulling Mesh Harness, an adaptation of their training harnesses, fits under the dog's "armpits" at a natural pressure point. When the dog pulls, the harness tightens and causes discomfort but not pain, so the dog stops pulling. The color choice is the same as for the leash. The harness comes in small, medium and large to fit dogs with neck sizes from 9 to 33 inches.

Shadow-Max's Jogger is a 6-foot adjustable leash with a snap at each end. One end attaches to an adjustable, quick-release waist belt that accommodates 24- to 40-inch human middles. The other end attaches to the dog's collar. Dog owners are often concerned that their dogs will get tangled up with the poles. Trail-savvy Chris Frado, president and executive director of the Cross-Country Ski Areas Association, who walks with two large dogs, reports, "I find that my dogs start out in front of me, but Nordic Walking allows me to have better stamina than them, and on the way home, they're beside me or sometimes a bit behind. The dogs figure out quickly where to be in relation to the poles and I've never had a problem." These products might solve the problem of walking both with your poles and your pooch, but it doesn't address the issue of a parent and a baby in a carriage or a toddler in a stroller. No one has yet devised a way to operate the poles and the parent-powered vehicle.

The gotta-haves for Nordic Walking are relatively few and relatively inexpensive. The wanna-haves are for those who like to dress up and to gear up with gadgetry.

Techniques

Years ago, in one of his routines, the late comedian George Carlin used to say, "There is a magazine for everything these days. Here's a new copy of *Walking* magazine. Check out page 12. It says, 'Put one foot in front of the other.'" *Walking* was a magazine ahead of its time—that time being now—but the publisher pulled the plug on it shortly before walking took off as a major health and fitness activity. Nordic Walking can be described in much the same way as that old Carlin joke: Put one foot in the other and one pole in front of the other in opposition —left foot/right pole and right foot/left pole.

Carlin always got a laugh for that one, but joking aside, while walking in general and Nordic Walking in particular are indeed simple, they are also profound in terms of benefits. The analogy that is often used to differentiate Nordic Walking from pole-less walking is the difference between four-wheel drive and two-wheel drive. Getting the most benefit from it in terms of calorie expenditure, cardiovascular conditioning and full-body muscle engagement requires an awareness of various elements of technique. David Downer, a long-time British Nordic Walking instructor, author, Nordic Walking eCommunity moderator and all-round authority on the topic, tells his students, "it's not walking unless it's Nordic Walking" And that is the benefit bonus in a nutshell.

Vive la Difference!

Nordic Walking is related to a several other walking activities but is different in important ways.

- **Walking/Nordic Walking**—This is pretty obvious. The former does not use poles. The latter requires them by definition.
- **ChiWalking**—Developed by running and walking coaches Danny and Katherine Dreyer, ChiWalking is a mind – body form of walking designed to strengthen, stabilize and energize the body while also relieving tension and focusing the mind. They counsel utilizing "Five Mindful Steps" to achieve lifelong health, improved fitness and tranquility.
- **Race-walking**—Race-walkers do not use poles either but employ a very specific technique that, in fact, is required in competition. One foot must be in contact with the ground at all times, with no loss of contact visible between steps. In other words, the heel of the front foot and the toe of the rear foot must simultaneously be touching the ground, even if briefly. Also, the advancing leg must be straight (not bent at the knee) from the heel strike until it is perpendicular to the ground, before bending and moving forward to the next step. In Nordic Walking, by contrast, the forward knee is slightly bent at each step. Also, race-walkers carry their arms low and close to the hips as they swing in opposition to the legs.
- **Power Walking**—A training regimen of walking fast, often for specific periods of time or predetermined distances, as part of a fitness routine, to increase endurance, burn calories or achieve other health goals. Walkers often have traditionally added weights, either on a weight belt or as wrist or hand weights, to increase the workload. Some are now beginning to use poles for the same result, which moves power walking into the Nordic Walking realm.
- **Mall Walking**—Indoor walking, generally in the long corridors of a shopping mall, often before the stores open, for health and fitness. Mall walking is especially popular in the Sunbelt belt in summer and the Frostbelt in winter. Seniors especially like smooth, obstacle-free mall floors. Many malls encourage walking with discreet distance markers, maps and even designated gathering spaces for groups of regulars. In 2009, the gigantic Mall of America in Minnesota became the first to reach out to Nordic Walkers. Mall walking predated Nordic Walking, and not all mall managers are as forward-thinking

as those at the Mall of America. Therefore, if you walk indoors with poles, always do so with rubber caps or booties to protect the floors from the metal tips—and also to prevent the tips from slipping on the hard surface.

- **Treadmill Walking**—Some types of treadmills are equipped with pole-like, pivoting handles that are moved forward and back while walking. This combined leg and arm motion approximates Nordic Walking using gym apparatus.

- **Nordic Track**—This branded, unmotorized device replicates the leg and arm motions of cross-country skiing indoors. It is related to Nordic Walking in name only, but the similar names do cause confusion among people who aren't clear on what Nordic Walking is all about. Nordic Track is an indoor substitute for an on-snow activity, while Nordic Walking is fitness walking with poles—outdoors.

- **Schigang or Skigang**—Pronounced "she-gahng," the original Nordic-skiing training exercise using longer cross-country poles to force the hands high in front in order to push forward. Cross-country skiers and ski teams in North America also developed similar energetic dry-land training drills, including energetic uphill and downhill training. This is also called "hill bounding" or "ski bounding."

- **Hiking with Poles/Trekking**—Hiking and Nordic Walking are related but different activities, and therefore, the specialized poles for each are truly different, both in design and in purpose. Nordic Walking poles have been described in Chapter 2. Hiking poles, which sometimes bear the same manufacturers' brands as Nordic Walking poles, are heavier and have grips and straps similar to ski poles. The main difference is their usage. While Nordic Walkers employ a very specific pole-plant position behind the forward foot to push off and propel themselves forward on fairly smooth ground, hikers usually plant their poles somewhere in front of the lead foot for stability, balance and control on steep and/or rough trails. Hikers do not push off on the back swing. The purpose of Nordic Walking poles (like Nordic Walking technique itself) is to increase energy expenditure and calorie burn, while trekking poles are designed to help hikers conserve energy. Finally, trekking or hiking poles are always made of aluminum for strength and durability in rugged conditions, while the most expensive Nordic Walking poles are made of carbon-fiber to be lightweight and somewhat flexible. While Nordic Walking poles can be either fixed-length/one-piece, modern hiking or trekking poles are always adjustable to accommodate sustained ascents or descents on steep, often rugged trails.

Learning to Nordic Walk: Class or Do-It-Yourself?

Technique wonks—those exercise and sports physiologists, trainers and coaches who develop and tweak the fine points of curriculum and certification requirements—have parsed the relatively simple activity of Nordic Walking into incredible detail. Some of them seem to have determined the ideal and very precise position of the hand when reaching forward or backward, the position of the head when striding, the placement of the feet with each step, the angle of the elbows, the degree to which the hand is opened on the backswing, and the rotation of the shoulders, almost measured down to the centimeter—which is only slightly facetious. These technique whizzes have determined the angle between the forearm and upper arm during the pole plant and the angle between the upper arm and the torso or ground at the apex of the backswing. And of course, they have determined the angle of the pole and the proper placement of the tip when the pole is planted. They are, in short, a determined lot—and each system seems slightly different from every other system. It is quite appropriate that these wizards have developed the highest level of ideal Nordic Walking technique, because that's what they do. In the process, reams have been written about these ultra-fine points. Illustrations have been drawn to diagram the precise position of the feet, arms and shoulders, and the sketches of the pole angle related to the ground, complete with the physics of where along the pole shaft the horizontal and vertical forces are exerted during the push-off phase of the pole plant.

For most of us, especially when we begin Nordic Walking, such minute details are way more than we need to know. We need to take a class, start walking, have an instructor or trainer correct the flaws that are counter to Nordic Walking's main benefits and etch enough technique into our muscle memory to be effective without being frustrated because we are concerned about too much detail. Maintaining a consistent pace and rhythm, propelling yourself forward with each pole plant, and enjoying the activity enough so that you will keep doing it will benefit you greatly. It is important to keep from becoming frustrated because you may end up feeling afraid you will do it incorrectly, which may keep you from going Nordic Walking. It can be argued that unless you are a competitive athlete looking for maximum training from each Nordic Walk or want to become an instructor, it is preferable to have less than perfect technique in favor of getting enough pleasure from Nordic Walking that you will continue doing it. If you are the sort who gets discouraged at anything less than perfection, try to scale down your ambitions.

All other things being equal, Nordic Walking is best learned in a class, because the most effective way to develop effective, if not necessarily "proper," technique is under the eye of a trainer or instructor. The better he or she is schooled—both in Nordic Walking technique and as a teacher—the more successful your class is likely to be. Marko Kantaneva is credited with developing the first system of pole walking in Europe and naming it Nordic Walking. It includes warm up exercises and drills and a specific skill-building progression to attain proper technique. With its origins as a summer regime for elite cross-country ski racers, the Europe-based International Nordic Walking Association (INWA) and its instructors approach Nordic Walking as a sport. It came as something of a surprise to pioneering European instructors that many of their early students were middle-age women who wanted to shape up rather than well-trained athletes who were already fit. The result was a scaling-down of the early phase of Nordic Walking instruction to make it more accessible to more people. The leadership of both the American Nordic Walking Association and the Canadian Nordic Walking Association have roots in Europe but developed slight variations on the INWA system, adding a New World viewpoint. Americans and Canadians have generally come to Nordic Walking from the fitness and wellness business. Other individual technique developers have come up with their own progressions. Of course, there is recognition that Nordic Walking provides competitive runners and other serious athletes with knee relief while not compromising their cardio conditioning. Maintaining aerobic fitness and stamina remains their main thrust, but other people are attracted to Nordic Walking in order to get fit, rather than to stay fit.

Because it has been around longer than other organizations, INWA has developed a more comprehensive curriculum with instructor training and certification at several levels. The INWA certification progression starts with a two-day, 16-hour basic instructor course and culminates in a master coach course that lasts at least 7 intense days. Many of the people seeking such a high level of certification have degrees in physiology or sports science. ANWA, still in its relative youth, began with a one-day, 8- to 10-hour certification course for the basic instructor level and has been adding higher levels as needed. At this writing, these are Certified Nordic Walking Basic Instructor, Certified Nordic Walking Advanced Instructor and Certified Professional Nordic Walking Instructor. Exterstrider, the first American walking pole company, finally introduced instructor training and certification two decades after its first walking poles came on the market. The Exerstriding Method is different from the others because Exerstrider poles have no strap. Instructor training launched in 2009. While the goals of organizations on both sides of the Atlantic ultimately converge, the attitudinal starting point is different—subtly so, perhaps, but worth tucking into the back of your mind.

The International Nordic Walking Association, with affiliated national organizations in various countries, was begun by Exel and certifies instructors in its techniques and progression using that brand of poles. North American instructors who have been certified by the American and Canadian Nordic Walking Associations usually use a major sponsor's poles but are able to develop, refine and tweak technique independently of a particular manufacturer. Additionally, some pole companies (for instance, the aforementioned Exerstrider, Fittrek, Keenfit, LEKI and SkiWalking) have developed their own programs and sometimes endorse instructors trained by other entities. They all train and in some fashion certify people to teach their versions, which vary slightly in the big picture. Some are derived from or are more closely related to the INWA/ANWA progression, but others were developed independently. American innovator Tom Rutlin introduced a distinctive strapless pole that he named Exerstrider in 1988 (which was some years before Exel and INWA) and developed a technique to go with it. Fittrek has allied itself with the fitness industry, with its progression recognized by the American Council on Exercise (ACE), Aerobics and Fitness Federation of America (AFFA) and Canadian Fitness Professionals (Can Fit Pro). Fittrek was also pro-active in encouraging footrace organizers to accept entrants with poles. (See Chapter 6 for more on races.) As noted in the Preface, no one method is necessarily better than the others, or absolute. Like the chocolate, vanilla or strawberry choice, it is more a matter of taste or training. Although the proponents of any one variation are reluctant to admit it, the similarities are, in fact, greater than the differences. The most important thing, really, is to sign up for a convenient class where you live or where you vacation, pick up a set of poles and begin Nordic Walking. Let's get started.

The ABCs of Nordic Walking Technique

The alphabet soup of certifying organizations (see Resources, page 159) can be confusing for beginners, so the intention of this section is to outline the teaching progressions of the leading family of international organizations, not to advocate any one approach over another. The closely related INWA/ANWA class formats in particular begin with short drills designed to make individuals comfortable with each other, the group and, most importantly, their poles.

Introductory classes therefore often start with what seems like silly stuff—almost playground games, in fact.. Examples? The instructor might have everyone place his or her poles in a circle and mill around within the circle without bumping into each other—and then mill around randomly and shake hands with every classmate encountered. There might be partner exercises like wordless Simon Says in which students are asked to mimic each others' moves with poles. There might be a Virginia Reel-type game requiring one person at a time to walk through a double line of classmates. There might be an exercise in which partners face each other and alternately push/pull a pair of poles, or do so with one partner behind the other. The instructor might ask everyone to find the balance point in the middle of the pole shaft and balance it on one finger. These exercises are physical warmups and also psychological ones, because even a class of strangers tends to loosen up when doing things that feel like children's games. So silly-seeming or not, these activities do serve a purpose.

Stretches and Warm Ups

Exercises and stretches with poles as props are often incorporated into group Nordic Walks. Some leaders do them at the beginning as a warm up, some at the end as a cool-down and some insert them in the middle of the session just for variety. Each exercise is usually repeated 10 to 20 times. The following are some of the more common ones you can do on your own.

Ankle rotations

With poles at your sides and slightly in front, lift one foot off the
ground and rotate the ankle clockwise and then counter-clockwise.
Repeat with the other foot.

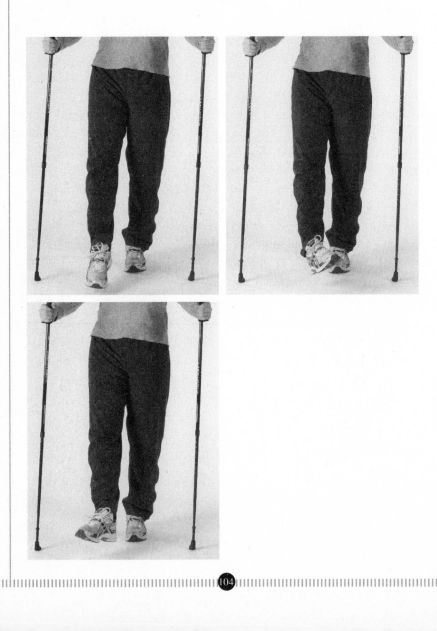

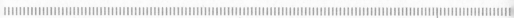

Hip stretches

Keeping your knees and arms straight but not locked, place your poles well in front of you and bend forward at the waist until your upper body is parallel to the ground. Keep your head in line with your body and your neck straight as you are stretching.

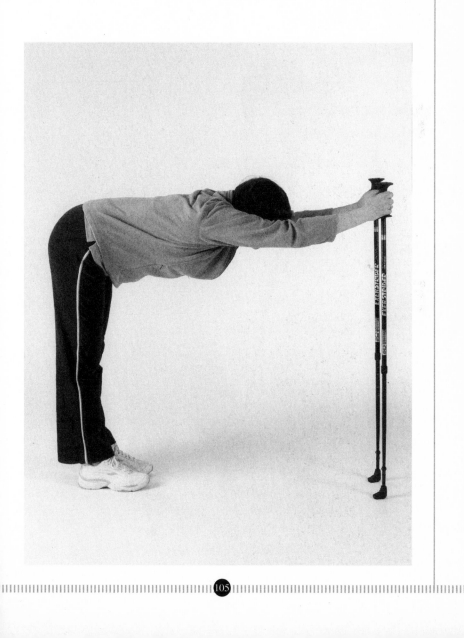

Leg stretches

Place your poles firmly at each side. Stretch one leg slightly in front of your body and alternately flex your foot (shown below) and point your toe. Repeat with the other leg.

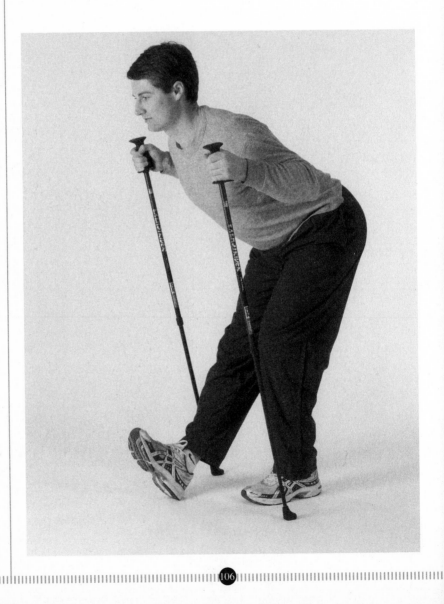

Lunges

Place your poles firmly in front of your body. Place one leg directly behind you, and sink down on the bended knee of the forward leg, with the rear leg remaining stretched behind you. Repeat with the other leg.

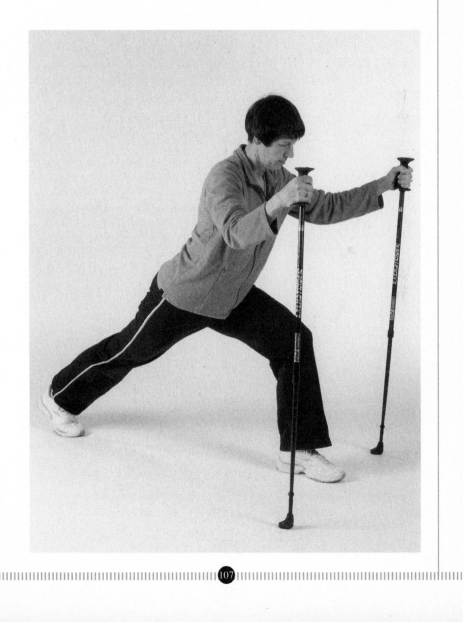

Quadricep stretches

Plant one or both poles firmly in front of your body, and hold it or them with one hand. Bend the opposite leg behind you, grasping your ankle with the hand on that side of the body, and pull the leg in toward your backside. Alternately, if your balance is good, stand on one leg, raise the other foot behind you, place one pole horizontally across the front of your ankle, and pull that foot toward you. Repeat with the other leg.

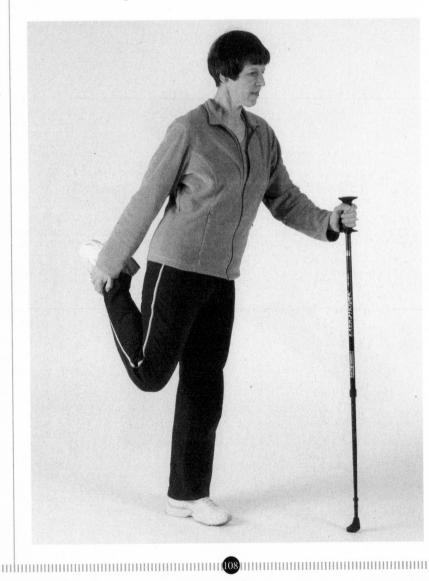

Shoulder and back stretches

With your poles planted in front of you, bend your knees, round your back, tuck in your tailbone, and contract your abdominal muscles (shown below). Then, reverse by straightening up, contracting your shoulder blades toward each other, and open your chest, keeping your pole tips in front of you but pulling the handles behind you approximately at hip level.

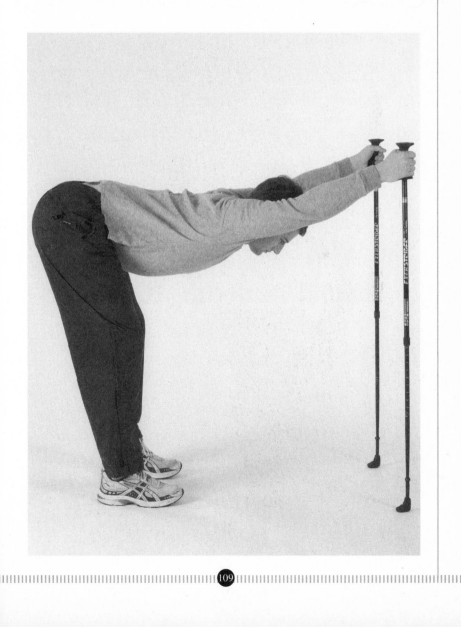

Side stretches

Hold the pole horizontally behind you, grab the shaft with both hands at a comfortable distance apart and alternately raise your left and right hands above your head, keeping both elbows slightly bent. A gentler alternative (shown below) is to grasp one pole in both hands, raise your arm in a V-shape and bend from side to side. An even gentler alternative is to hold a pole in front of you with your arms straight and bend at the waist, directly to the side. In all versions, pull your rib cage up and away from your hips, contracting your abdominal muscles as you bend to the side. Repeat on the other side.

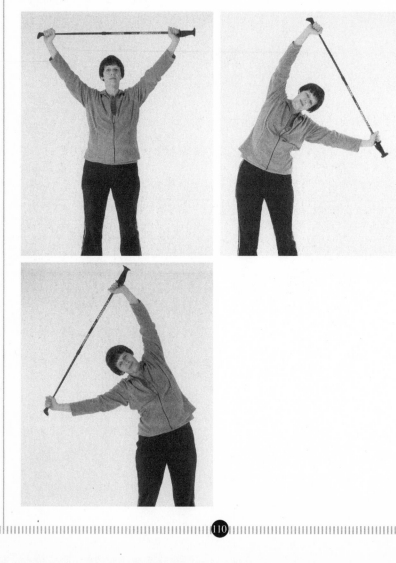

Squats

Holding one pole shoulder high behind the body, bend the knees and lower the body, tail first, as if to sit down in a chair. Straighten the knees and come up to standing.

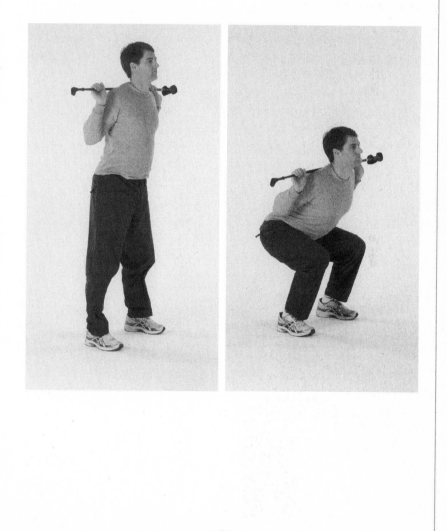

Upper arm and shoulder stretches

Grasp one pole vertically behind you and close to the body, bending both elbows. Pull down with the lower arm. Then, reverse by straightening the upper arm and bending the elbow of the lower arm and pulling upward. Repeat on the other side.

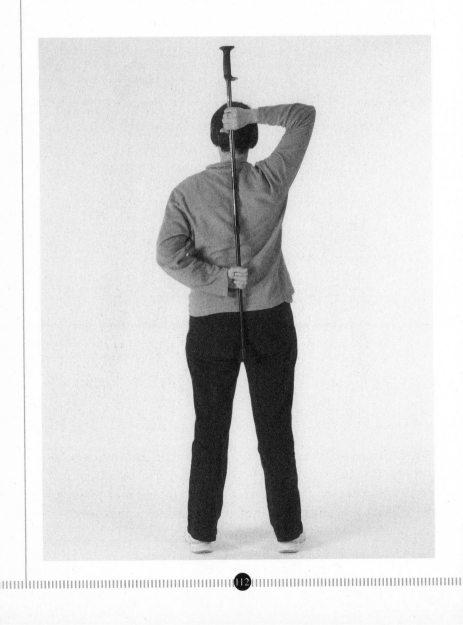

Waist rotations

Place a pole behind your neck, across your shoulders, and rotate at the waist, alternately left and right.

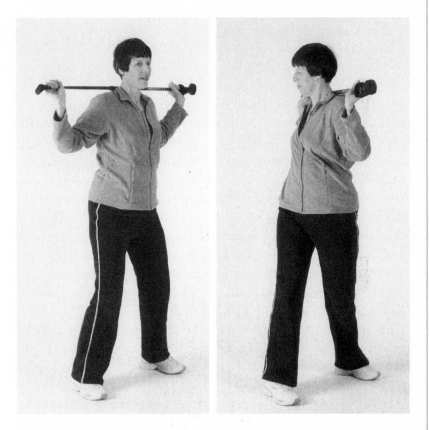

Note: Classes and group walks generally include such exercises, but in truth, once they start going out on their own, the vast majority of Nordic Walkers simply start walking—at a moderate pace to warm up—without doing these exercises every time they step out with their poles.

Finding an Instructor

In much of Europe, Nordic Walking instruction is common in cities and resorts alike—and, in fact, some countries' national health plans subsidize fitness-walking instruction. In North America, you have to look a little harder to find a trained instructor. Nordic Walking sessions might be based out of running or footwear retail stores, fitness centers, wellness programs, outdoor clubs, private gyms and studios, senior centers, YMCAs and YWCAs, recreation programs and more. Some personal trainers have also taken on Nordic Walking as one of their specialties and promote it locally. One good way to find classes or instructors is on the Internet. Nordic Walking associations' Web sites provide lists of instructors they have certified. Pole makers' sites (including www.nordicwalker.com, www.nordicwalking.com, www.leki.com, www.fittrek.com, www.keenfit.com, and www.skiwalk.com) also list instructors who have taken their training. These names are organized geographically by state, so it's fairly easy to narrow the search down to your area. These Web sites sometimes also include a calendar of events listing with upcoming class schedules. As Nordic Walking's popularity picks up, these sites' search functions will surely become more refined—but also harder to keep up-to-date as more instructors are trained. Another, arguably more productive, place to check is the activities calendars of hometown newspapers; local Web sites may also include classes and contact information. While association and manufacturer sites provide contact information, local resources also give details of start dates, costs and locations for upcoming Nordic Walking classes.

You can often find a free or very inexpensive local introductory session, probably just an hour or an hour and a half, that covers just the fundamentals and generally includes the use of poles during the session. Brief as that seems, such a session really is enough to get the basics. Because pole length is crucial to Nordic Walking, instructors start by helping everyone adjust his or her poles to the proper length or select the right ones from a quiver of fixed-length poles. The instructors also show how the hands are put through the straps properly (some brands are more intuitively designed than others) even before taking those first steps. At the end of such an introductory session, some people will be striding confidently and rhythmically, while others will still be trying to get it right.

Some instructors offer a series of classes or group walks, with or without the use of poles included in the fee. Often scheduled weekly at the same time and same meeting place, these group walks are ideal for companionship and ongoing technique refinement. Instructors with a background as fitness instructors or personal trainers in health clubs, gyms or recreation centers might institute a punch card system that encourages new Nordic Walkers to return because they have prepaid additional sessions.

Kerry A. Wiley on Nordic Walking to "Best Live Her Life"

"I have a diagnosis of Spastic Cerebral Palsy and have used some form of a cane or crutch for the past 25 years. Spastic Cerebral Palsy is merely a clinical diagnostic term to define challenges I have to walk. I use whatever tools I can to best live my life and the Nordic Poles have been one of those tools. To treat the problem, doctors had me switch walking devices. I was using Canadian Crutches and they were not working for me. They were heavy and cumbersome and I was prone to falls with them. Then I started to develop pain in my hands, arms and shoulders, all of which resulted from overuse of the canes and crutches. Rosie Breault of Kennfit sent walking poles to me. She recognized the benefits that I could gain from using the Keenfit Walking Poles—and they changed my life. With Nordic Walking poles, I used my legs, more than my arms, to stand and the pressure on my arms, hands and shoulders was less. I can stand easily with the poles. I have better posture and can pick up my feet better. In October 2007, when I took the poles to my personal trainer, Jason Berner at Plaza Fitness (at Stuyvesant Plaza in Albany, New York), he said, 'I want you using these poles full time.' The Keenfit Walking Poles have given me more freedom. They have been tools that have improved my gait and have allowed me to do what I have never done before."

Anyone with a particular physical challenge would need to undertake Nordic Walking with a physical therapist who understands how poles can help, or with a personal trainer who is experienced in working with people who have disabilities—either chronic or temporary (including recovery from joint replacement surgery).

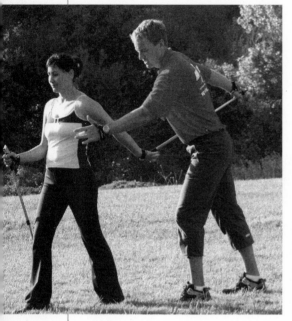

Learning Styles & Teaching Styles

Different learning styles identified by psychologists and educators beginning in the 1970s that are relevant when you start out in a Nordic Walking class include:

• If you are a visual learner, you will benefit most from watching an instructor demonstrate proper technique and imitating it. Instructional CDs, DVDs or videos are also most useful for visual learners.
• Some people also seem to be "visualizing learners," who benefit from "seeing" themselves doing something before they actually do it.
• If you are an auditory learner, you will benefit from an instructor's explanation because words and phrases that help describe the correct technique will implant it in your mind. It will be helpful to be told, for instance, that the forward position of your arm should be in the "handshake position" or that your arms should move "like pump handles" and be positioned close to your body and parallel to each other "like railroad tracks."
• If you are a kinesthetic learner, you will pick up proper technique by trying, adjusting to an instructor's error detection and correction, and knowing what proper technique feels like when you "get it."
• If you learn by processing written words and putting them into practice, this book and other more detailed descriptions of Nordic Walking will be key learning tools for you.

Successful instructors, not just in Nordic Walking but in other fitness and physical activities as well, identify their students' learning styles and tailor their teaching to their class and the individuals in it. If one thing doesn't work for a particular student, they will try something else. Some instructors like to teach perfect form from the beginning, even if not all students can achieve it. Others prefer roughly correct form and then help students refine it once they begin the activity. In any case, characteristics of effective instruction include:

- Demonstration and explanation of proper technique.
- Error detection and appropriate correction when a student is making a technical error
- Injury prevention
- Positive reinforcement whenever a student is progressing and improving
- Encouragement even when a student is having problems
- The ability to dissect a movement in order to isolate just part of it for demonstration, correction or explanation
- The ability to verbally describe the desired movements, using imagery when necessary, to help students understand the goal of that instruction phase
- Weaving a review of what has been learned into the next phase
- The energy to keep a class moving and enjoyable for those who catch on quickly as well as for those who need a little more time

How well a class learns and how effectively an instructor teaches play out in infinite variations. Nordic Walking classes tend to be limited in size by the number of available pole sets, but consider that a beginning instructor who has just passed a basic certification class probably has all he or she can handle with half-a-dozen students. An experienced instructor who has led large aerobics, Pilates, yoga or other fitness classes can usually effectively teach the fundamentals to about 15 new Nordic Walkers.

The Class Society: What to Expect

Visualize this: You and your classmates have your poles properly adjusted, with your hands in the straps (except for strapless Exerstriders),

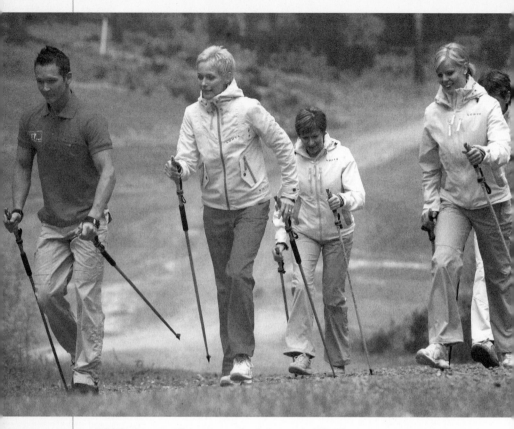

and the straps also properly tightened. The instructor gets the group with a series of warm ups and stretches, soon to be followed by a simple walk without poles. If you are taking those first steps on asphalt or pavement, you will probably have the paws or caps on the pole tips, but many instructors like beginners to start on grass, on a smooth, unpaved trail or even on wet sand using the metal tips. Although many classes start with a series of warm up exercises, others get right into the introductory phase of Nordic Walking and add the exercises later. Common exercises are covered above on pages 104-113.

In either case, before you even begin the preliminary poling action itself, the instructor will have you stand tall, leading with your rib cage and with your head held high. You will be asked to begin walking comfortably, letting your arms swing naturally with each step. Whether a class starts with a simple walk without poles, or with students carrying their poles to get a sense of their weight and balance, the instructor might ask you to notice the rhythmic swing of your arms, with left arm/right leg and right arm/left leg moving in opposition. Cross-country skiers find this a natural dry-land version of the diagonal stride of classical Nordic ski technique.

Again in either case, you will probably be told to concentrate on using the full mobility of your feet with each step, planting your heel, keeping your weight centered or even distributed toward the outside of the feet, rolling through the balls of your feet and pushing off from the toes. One foot is always in contact with the ground. Never lock your knees, but rather, keep them very lightly flexed.

The next step is usually holding your poles loosely in your hands and letting the tips drag on the ground behind you. After a short time, the instructor will ask you to again begin using your arms in opposition to your legs, bringing your arm forward but not higher than waist level with each step. Some instructors want students to begin touching the pole tips lightly onto the ground at the beginning of each backswing right away. Once you start using the poles, you should be keeping the pole shafts at about a 45-degree angle to the ground so that when your hand moves forward, the pole tip does not pass the plane in front of your leading foot or your body.

As you become comfortable with this motion, the next stage is to begin pushing or pressuring on the strap. When you do this, you will feel yourself using the muscles of your arms, shoulders and upper body. You will also feel the pole tips engage with each step. When this becomes comfortable, you will begin actively pressuring or pushing off, starting at the apex of the forward swing, using pressure on the strap to transmit force through the pole to the ground. Except with Exerstrider poles, your instructor will direct you to open your hand on each backswing as your arm passes your hip line. As your arm comes forward, you will catch the pole grip again as it passes the plane of your body. At the high point of the back swing, the arm should be fairly straight, and the pole should be an extension of the arm with the tip a few inches off the ground. Automatic rotation of the shoulder accompanies each arm movement. Therefore, you will be working right arm/right shoulder/left leg, left arm/left shoulder/right leg along with the backswing/open hand, forward swing/closed hand, effecting a full range of motion in your shoulder joints. Ideally, you will plant the pole solidly and firmly without bouncing, wiggling the tip or paw around or grinding it into the ground. You don't want to drag the pole on the ground either, nor should you fling it up in the air on the backswing.

The goal is to use your poles to propel yourself forward with each pole plant. The coordination for the "grab and go" or "grasp and/or release" or "catch and release" aspect—whatever your instructor calls it—is one of the more difficult aspects of Nordic Walking for many beginners to get the hang of. Therefore, as you plant each pole, your hand should open up during the propulsion phase and close as you "retrieve" it during the forward swing. In other words, as you move your arm forward, grasp the grip lightly so that you will be ready to plant the pole, pressure it to the ground and propel yourself forward at the next step. A vise-like grip of the pole grip is never necessary—and in fact would be tiring. Just grasp your poles lightly and comfortably with each step. The padded straps are affixed near the tops of the handles in order to help your hand stay in the proper position and prevent your poles from getting away from you. It is important to practice it and get it right, because an ungrasped pole (during the forward swing) is a loose pole. It is the Nordic Walking equivalent of a loose cannon and can trip you up if it detours between your legs as you are striding along. Ouch!

Once you have become comfortable and have found your rhythm, you will automatically lengthen your stride, lean your upper body forward slightly with your head up and your eyes looking ahead to see where you are going, not down at your feet, and you will find yourself picking up speed. Congratulations. You are now a Nordic Walker!

Marek Zalewski's Thoughts on Technique Variations

Zalewski, a Nordic Walking instructor in northern Virginia, who founded Nordic Walking US, has taught, practiced and long pondered the intricacies of straight versus bent elbows and knees.

"By far the most important issue is to simply go out there and walk, even if it isn't in a 'prescribed' style. For those who teach Nordic Walking, those who race and those who want to look their best out there, the fine technique and style points might be more important. Personally, I used to walk with a bent arm, thinking that this contributed to a better triceps workout. A bit later, I became convinced that the straight arm stroke contributes more to a full-body core/trunk workout, while still providing a good triceps exercise. I have never felt comfortable with the fully straight, rigid arm position. Therefore, my preferred technique is a bit more relaxed and fluid. I tend to keep my arm a bit straighter than some people but not quite as straight as others. Frankly, I haven't seen anyone walking with a completely straight arm. Although I do recognize the speed benefits of the straight leg race-walking technique, unless I am racing and/or trying to beat a personal record, I tend to walk with a soft knee, relaxed gait and usually in tempo with the music from my MP3 player actually propelling me along. I also believe that this sort of a more fluid and less forceful motion is safer on the joints and muscles in the long run.

"In short, I tell people: Go out there. Have fun. Exercise your body and your mind, and do not overly concern yourselves with the fine points of technique. Everybody has a slightly different style of walking, running, skiing and Nordic Walking. Wouldn't it be funny to see a group of Nordic Walkers walking in exactly the same style and in absolutely perfect synch?"

Making the Right Moves

As indicated earlier, different manufacturers and organizations suggest slight technique variations. People respond to different word pictures. Again, to teach yourself the basic moves or to reinforce what you have learned in class, look over the 10 ANWA-style tips for Nordic Walking Basics, LEKI's 5 technique tips, Exel's 4 tips and Fittrek's 7 tips, and see what resonates with you. The very fine points of pole use vary. According to some schools of Nordic Walking thought, particularly the European INWA methodologists and their philosophical/physiological offspring, the elbow should be slightly bent as if ready to shake someone's hand at the forward-most arm position. According to others, notably Exerstrider's Tom Rutlin, the elbow should be nearly straight—not rigid, but more straight than not. In the early days of Nordic Walking, proper technique called for keeping the hand open longer. At this writing, the ideal seems to be to grab the pole quickly and plant it as soon as the hand is at its forward-most position. Some Nordic Walking pioneers still keep their hands open longer, and Exerstrider users do not really open them at all.

Ten Basic Tips from ANWA

One of the appeals of Nordic Walking is its inherent simplicity. Whether you want to try to teach yourself, perhaps with the help of a DVD or on line film or guidance from a more experienced companion, or review what you have learned in a class, below are the fundamentals of Nordic Walking technique, as taught by ANWA-certified instructors. These slightly academic-sounding written descriptions of, and instructions for, Nordic Walking technique often use many words to describe nuanced movements that are really best learned from a trained instructor—someone who can demonstrate, watch you as you begin learning the most effective technique, correct large or small errors, reinforce what you are doing correctly and help you refine your movements until they become automatic. This section is therefore meant as an adjunct to in-person instruction, not as a substitute for it. It is intended to present you with an idea as to what to expect in a Nordic Walking class, and as reinforcement for what you have learned once you have taken a class, not as a substitute for learning from an instructor.

1. Find a short practice route, either on a paved path (with rubber paws, caps or booties on the pole tips) or on grass or an unpaved trail (without paws).

2. Set your poles aside, and walk briskly around this route, letting your arms swing naturally. Notice that your left foot and right arm move forward and back together, as do your right foot and left arm. This natural, oppositional stride is the foundation of Nordic Walking.

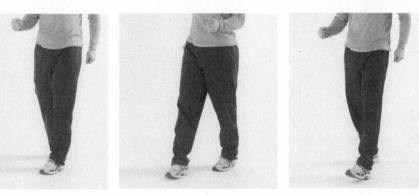

3. Pick up your poles and repeat your route, letting the pole tips drag behind you. Stand tall and lead with your rib cage.

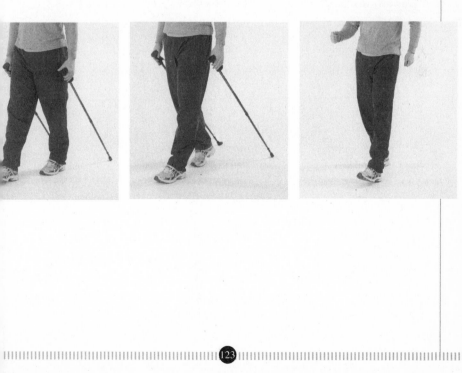

4. Repeat your route again, allowing the tip of the pole in the forward hand to touch the ground lightly.

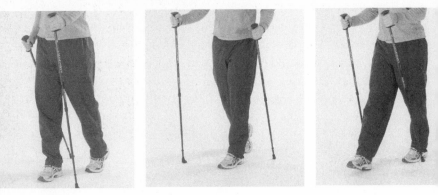

5. Be aware of what you are doing with your feet. Start each step by applying the heel to the ground, then roll through the full length of each foot and finish each step by pressing forward from the ball of the foot, and then the toes.

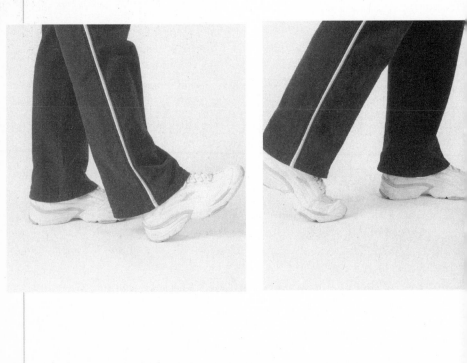

6. Be aware of what you are doing with your hands. As your hand passes the plane of your body on the backswing, open your fingers to release the pole grip. As your hand passes the plane of your body while moving forward, catch the pole grip. *(Author's note: The exception is Exerstrider, shown in bottom photos. Because it is strapless, the hand does not open.)*

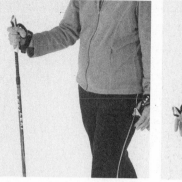
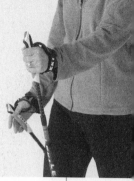

LEKI

7. With each step, begin pressuring your pole tip against the ground behind the heel of your forward foot and ahead of the toe of the back foot. At the same time, push your pole tip against the ground by pressing the heel of your hand against the pole strap.

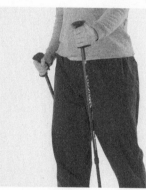

Exerstrider

8. As you become comfortable with the two concurrent but alternating aspects of Nordic Walking (pole plant/pole release, left foot/right arm and right foot/left arm), begin pressuring the pole tip against the ground to feel your shoulder and torso muscles engaging, providing a full-body workout. This will happen automatically.

9. Allow your upper body to rotate lightly and naturally. It is not a twist, but a subtle rotation.

10. When you become comfortable, you will find yourself moving more easily, more dynamically and more rhythmically, picking up speed and increasing your endurance.

Four Steps in Exel's Progressive Walking Technique

The following four stages are outlined in Exel's Progressive Nordic Walking Technique, below. Read them all, let them sink in and remember that some words may resonate with you more than others. You can even practice these moves indoors if you like, with imaginary poles, just to get the cadence. Then, take your poles outside and walk in a natural stride with arms and legs moving in opposition (right arm/left leg, left arm/right leg), first just carrying the poles, then dragging them, moving on to gently tipping the ground and finally planting the poles. With confidence, begin propelling yourself forward with each pole plant. Here are the same essential steps as described in the Exel progression:

1. Initial Phase of Nordic Walking Cadence
- The walker's right arm is forward and slightly bent with the pole held at an angle.
- The left hand is past the line of the pelvis, and the left arm extends back during pole thrust.
- The right leg is extended at the ankle as it pushes off the ground. The left leg is forward with the heel making contact with the ground to begin a new stride.

2. Pole Thrust Stage
- The right arm's pole thrust and the left leg thrust take place more or less simultaneously.
- The fists of the hands pass by one another slightly in front of the body, and the right-hand pole thrust begins as soon as it passes the line of the pelvis. At the same time, the left arm swings under and forward with the fist and pole grip foremost.
- The right leg is slightly bent at the knee as it moves level with the left leg. The left leg and the pole in the right hand share the weight and the pressure of each stride.

3. Pole Thrust Stage
- The pole thrust is completed as the right arm extends itself fully. To effectively complete arm extension the palm of the hand opens out

slightly and the final thrust is made via the pole strap.

- At the same time the left fist and pole grip lift slightly upwards and forward as the arm bends at the elbow.
- The left leg is extended at the ankle as it thrusts off the ground while the right leg is forward with the heel strike beginning a new stride.

4. Final Stage of Pole Thrust

- The right hand's pole thrust ends with the palm of the hand opening out and the arm almost fully extended. The left arm's pole thrust is beginning.
- The left leg begins its effort, and the weight transfers to the right leg. The body leans markedly forward.

Technique Tips from LEKI

The following step-by-step technique recommendations are from LEKI, which makes adjustable poles. Other organizations and manufacturers offer similar but not identical sequences:

- **Get Adjusted**: Pole height is directly related to preventing overuse injuries! Adjustable poles accommodate most heights. To measure, place your hands in the straps. The rubber tips should be adjacent to your heels. Stand in good posture, and drop the hands forward in the straps to lengthen through the elbows. The wrists should be lower than the elbows.
- **Coordinate Your Effort**: Nordic walking takes some coordination. It's called an "opposing arm and leg swing." It's the way we're supposed to walk, but most people have forgotten to involve their upper bodies! Spend the first several minutes, if not several hours, simply getting used to walking with poles using your coordination. Hands should be relaxed. The farther your lead hand comes out in front, the more you'll feel how that tip engages to propel you forward.
- **Stand Tall**: Postural strength is a primary benefit of Nordic Walking. As you walk, try to keep the bottom of your chin level with the surface. This small skill helps to balance your head weight more appropriately over the rest of your skeleton, allowing you to reap optimal benefits from your Nordic walking experiences!

- **Longer Is Better**: Fitness benefits are maximized with a long arm technique which inspires a longer gait. If you find yourself bending excessively at the elbows, lighten your grips and lengthen your arms. Movement comes from the shoulders, not the elbows!
- **Take Your Time**: Changing your stride takes time, so remember to have fun—and don't think too hard!

Seven from Fittrek

Fittrek founder Dan Barrett's refinement of Nordic Walking technique includes what might be called sub-techniques for particular situations. From easiest to most challenging, they are:

- **First Steps for Beginners:** Place the pole tips behind your feet and relax your arms. Begin walking with hands open, allowing the straps to hold the poles. After a couple of minutes of dragging the poles, swing your arms in a natural walking motion, opposite arm moving forward with opposing leg, with hands remaining open. Once this motion feels comfortable, exaggerate the arm motion on the forward swing, gently grasp the poles and push off with the trailing arm. Now you're Nordic Walking! The next step is to select the technique or techniques best suited for your goals.
- **Nordic Walking/Full Power:** Derived from dry land training techniques from Nordic skiing, this technique recruits the most muscles for those seeking to increase the intensity of their fitness-walking. It allows for maximum push-off with the poles. In optimum conditions the pushing arm can be fully extended until in line with the pole behind body. This technique is best for soft terrain where the poles really bite. It is not recommended for individuals with lower body concerns such as "bad" knees. Some of our following techniques are better suited for unloading or stabilizing the lower body. To learn this technique, begin with the…

  …Hands Open Style. Gently grasp handles, lift the tips a few inches off the ground when bringing arms forward. Do not swing the pole tips forward. The tips should plant about 10-20 inches behind the lead foot. Arms should remain almost straight. On soft terrain where push-off is increased, hand can release from the poles at the end phase of the push-off.

- **Nordic Walking/Standard:** Fittrek calls this Standard because it feels the most natural for most walkers. It is best used when walking at a relatively faster pace. For example, when Nordic Walking with someone with a longer stride, they may use Full Power and you can use Standard, with a faster step rate. Standard is also good to use when the terrain doesn't allow for aggressive push-offs and longer pole lengths. To learn this technique, begin with Full Power, then increase the bending of the elbow until the arm movement is about fifty-fifty between the shoulders and elbows.

- **Nordic Walking/Fast:** To move even faster you must step faster. By using a relatively shorter pole length and moving the arms primarily at the elbows, an individual can increase their step rate. The Fast technique allows people with shorter leg length to Nordic Walk with people with longer legs and greater stride length.

- **Nordic Walking/On-Road:** When Nordic Walking on asphalt or concrete, the traction tread tips increase the friction (or bite) of the pole tips, but not to the same level as the sharp off-road tips on soft terrain. To compensate for the decreased push-off, you must increase the forward motion off the poles. In this technique, the pole tip swings forward so it can be planted beside the lead foot. The arm motion is just like reaching out to shake someone's hand. The push-off phase can be maintained until the pole tip loses traction, or arm and pole can be extended with pole tip leaving ground.

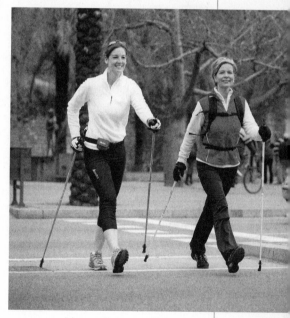

- **Nordic Walking/Off-Road:** This technique is derived from the common use of poles on the trail where unloading tired or overloaded legs are a priority. This style is great for Nordic Walkers with lower body orthopedic concerns or rehabilitation applications because it reduces leg load and impact with every step. In this style, the poles function like a second pair of legs. The tips plant evenly with the opposite foot on each step. Keep arm motion to a minimum and allow poles to swing into position. Gentle pressure downward on the poles "lifts" the body up, unloading the legs.

- **Nordic Walking/Up-hill:** Keep poles on a positive angle and push off to power yourself up the hill.

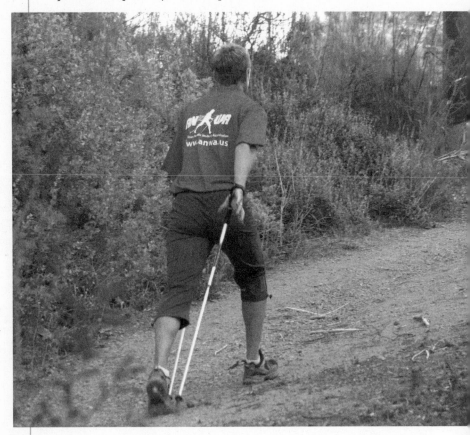

- **Nordic Walking/Down-hill:** When going down steep declines, the primary use of the poles is to minimize pressure on the knees. If it is a long descent, poles should be adjusted to a longer position. The steeper the decline, the longer the poles should be. Maintain opposing arm/leg movement as in all other techniques. Keep the arm movement limited and press down on the leading pole to unload the leading leg.

The placement of the pole tip in relation to the feet also varies. Most techniques call for the pole to be placed on a plane between the leading foot and the back foot. Fittrek's Barrett builds different pole positions into the specific variations that he developed. Pete Edwards, founder of SkiWalking and developer of the American Nordic Walking System, believes that the pole tip should be planted on a line with the heel of the leading foot. All of these styles, no matter how the details vary, are greatly beneficial for Nordic Walkers, provided that they engage their upper bodies and push off robustly with their poles to propel themselves forward and get that aerobic and calorie-burning bonus over walking without poles.

The Wayward Wind

If you are walking on a windy day, particularly in a cross-wind, the risk of being tripped up by a loose pole is greater. The stronger the wind, the greater the potential problem. Controlling your poles with a definite grip as soon as you begin the forward swing cuts the hazard, which can be likened to the Nordic Walker's equivalent of an aircraft hitting windshear. Some experienced Nordic Walkers grip the poles more solidly, shorten their steps and/or plant their poles more vertically or farther forward in windy conditions. Others simply stay indoors until the wind dies down!

Handling Hills, Slippery Surfaces and Other Terrain Challenges

Most people have to reduce their walking speed on uphill sections of the route and prudently slow down on downhill portions. The tactics are built into the Fittrek catechism. Instructors who subscribe to other methods introduce their classes to handling uphill and downhill portions of a trail. They often point out that uphills require a slight forward lean, a more forceful push-off from the ball of the foot and a longer stride, achieved by moving the front arm farther forward. Downhills require a firmly upright body position (or even one with the weight shifted slightly back), as well as shortened steps, a deeper

Rhea Kontos on Her Commitment to Nordic Walking

For some people, Nordic Walking is love at first step. That's the way it was for Rhea Kontos of Prior Lake, MN. She read about Nordic Walking, signed up for classes and went straight to becoming certified as an instructor. Her 'Nordic Walk This Way' program is active in the Twin Cities area, where she introduces newcomers to walking with poles in summer and on snow.

"I have been Nordic Walking since May '07 and have enjoyed ever minute of it. I can't say that about any other exercise program that I have been involved in. I have benefited both physically and socially. I found myself intrigued by an article back in April '07 that led me to picking up some poles and trying it for myself. Before that I was a casual jogger and my knees were not enjoying that pounding. Right away I could tell the benefits of Nordic Walking, and being an online junkie, I started investigating it further. Lo and behold ANWA was coming to my area very soon, so I signed on for the Basic Instructor class in Nov '07 to learn from [ANWA master trainer] Gottfried Kürmer. Soon after that I started instructing mostly via Community Education venues.

"With ANWA training I became better at the technique to maximize the positive affects and became certified to teach others. Initially, I became aware that my posture improved. Next came an overall feeling of better cardiovascular health, followed by general toning, especially in the biceps and triceps. Never have my arms looked this toned. And I didn't have to go to the club to achieve this. No waiting in lines, no sharing others' sweaty dumbbells. Nordic Walking outside is the best. However, one can walk indoors as well. Being from Minnesota, I have found plenty of public buildings to Nordic Walking inside.

"With training, I have been pleasantly surprised with the social interaction that comes with Nordic Walking. It is one of the few exercises you can enjoy and still maintain a conversation. Finding and maintaining these friendships has been a motivating factor for myself and many of those that I have trained. I trained a small group, with a super-senior couple who were eager to learn. They stuck with the training, joining me and others in many outdoor walks. I invited them to join me for the 5K Walk in the Birkie Trek in Hayward, WI. Not knowing what they were in for, they signed up and participated. They completed the hilly 5K in just an hour. It was their first 5K ever—and not their last. They also tried snowshoeing with me leading the way. I still Nordic Walk with this couple and actually quite miss them when they can't make it."

bend of the downhill knee and feet placed farther apart for increased stability. While Nordic Walking technique typically does not use poles to support the body, it is practical to do so on steep downhills. Particularly on an unpaved path, you'll probably want to slow down on downhill sections until you are comfortable with your footing. If the slope is really steep, you can plant your poles, either one at a time or simultaneously, in front of your body to help support yourself and eliminate the backswing until you are on level ground again. This interrupts the Nordic Walking rhythm, but it's better to be safe and secure than slipping and sorry.

Double poling, a move used less in Nordic Walking than in cross-country skiing or hiking/trekking, means planting and releasing both poles simultaneously. Skiers use it for power and speed. Hikers and trekkers use it to help on steep uphill pulls or to brace themselves on steep downhills, especially on rough terrain. If you find yourself on a steep trail, you can experiment with double poling for security and balance, both on the ascent and on the descent.

In fall, when dry or damp leaves cover sidewalks and roadways, you might find your poles slipping if you are using the rubber paws. You can either remove them and live with the clicking of the metal tips against the concrete or asphalt, or press back less aggressively until you reach clean pavement. Other suggestions are to try planting the poles a couple of inches farther forward than usual, (reducing the range of the backswing) or holding the poles more upright (more vertically) than you generally would. Sometimes simply slowing down the pace reduces slippage. When you encounter such conditions, experiment a little to see what works.

Rainy or snowy surfaces present another "opportunity" for the pole to slip. First, if you Nordic Walk in a wet area, make sure that the paws are not so worn that there is no traction left. You wouldn't drive on bald tires, so you shouldn't be Nordic Walking on slick surfaces with bald booties either. If they are in good shape, you can try pressuring more firmly on your poles. When pavement is wet or snowy, use your paws or caps. If the booties are bare-treaded, slow down, shorten your steps, push off less assertively, and adjust your entire poling motion forward—that is, plant your pole farther ahead than normal and shorten your backswing. Some paw designs provide more traction than others (see Chapter 2). If rain freezes on pavement, remove the paws or caps so that the metal tip can dig in to provide some traction—and perhaps slow down even more. LEKI makes a replacement paw with little metal spikes to provide additional traction, and you can also slip YakTrax, STABILicers or other devices onto your shoes or boots. If the precipitation comes in the form of snow, use the metal tips and also underfoot traction aids—and if it gets even deeper so that you sink several inches, add pole baskets and consider snowshoeing instead of walking. In any case, you have to find out what works by doing it—carefully—under these challenging conditions.

Summarizing Techniques

Perhaps your head is spinning from many words used to describe what are variations on the same basic technique. If you can't take it all in and want just one short piece of motivational advice to get you started, read this one. Before they even start, some people seem to get so hung up on the "right" technique and the "best" equipment that they don't dare take their poles out of the house. Don't be one of them. For most people, under most circumstances, Nordic Walking can be a fairly simple activity with fairly simple equipment. Get a good pair of shoes that fit right and are suitable for the weather where you live. The best choices (but not the only choices) are Nordic Walking shoes, walking shoes or trail-running shoes. Get a pair of poles (one-piece or adjustable) that feel comfortable in your hand and are within your budget—and, if one-piece, are the right length for your height.

Take a workshop or class if available (check with your local sporting goods or running store, YMCA/YWCA, hospital wellness/rehab program, rec center, adult education program or, if you are of an age, senior center). If you do sign up for a class, the instructor or coach will guide you through those first steps, including the proper angle for your elbow, the placement of the pole tip where it touches the ground, whether to open your hand on the backswing and if so, when to do so, and all sorts of other minutiae, according to his or her training. If you can't find a class, wing it. It's better than leaving your poles inside. So watch a DVD and try to emulate it. Get a trainer, friend or partner with some fitness/PE/sports savvy to compare what you are doing with what the pro on the DVD is doing.

The basics are rather intuitive. Follow the (usually illustrated) instructions that came with your poles to hold them effectively. Avoid clamping your hands around the pole handles in a death grip, but hold them loosely and comfortably. Start walking, moving your arms and legs in opposition (right arm/left leg, left arm/right leg), just as in regular walking. Place each pole tip on the ground somewhere on a line between the heel of your forward foot and the toe of your back foot. Press down and back on the pole lightly as you "move through" the step. As you gain confidence, lengthen your stride, pick up the pace and put more pressure on the pole. For some people, this confidence comes in a few minutes, for some in a few hours and for some only after a number of walks.

Then, if you choose, you can go beyond that. Refine your technique by reading an instructional book, revisiting instructional DVDs or looking harder for an instructor—perhaps taking a vacation or weekend escape someplace with a Nordic Walking program. As you progress, tweak your equipment if you wish. Get some advanced training. Join a group. Start a group.

Once you get into the Nordic Walking habit, you will find yourself striding along, enjoying the feeling of freedom and reveling in the knowledge that you are doing something good for yourself, even if you aren't using the "best" poles, the most prestigious footwear brand or the most flawless technique. After all, Nordic Walking for health, wellness and pleasure is not a figure skating, diving or gymnastics competition. No one is going to mark you down for technical flaws. No one is going to be concerned with which model of which brand pole you are using, or what logo is on your footwear.

Unless you are out to become a certified instructor or serious race competitor, don't get so hung up on the minutiae that you are reluctant to begin Nordic walking and so worried about the details that you can't enjoy the activity.

How Long a Walk is Long Enough?

A common question from beginning Nordic Walkers is, "How long (or how far) should I walk?" There is no one-size-fits-all answer, because of course, it depends on each individual's starting point. A person who has been fitness-walking without poles or a runner who is taking up Nordic Walking can walk farther and faster the first time he or she starts using poles than someone who has been sedentary. Since distance

DVDs Can Help

Some pole companies have produced instructional and motivational DVDs demonstrating and explaining the basics of Nordic Walking. They can serve as a good introduction or a good refresher, often supplementing guidance from an instructor or trainer. DVDs available at this writing include:

- Boomyah has an instructional video, free with each set of poles.
- Exel delivers a beginner DVD, free with each set of poles.
- Exerstrider has a 31-minute instructional video; clips are on the company's Web site (www.exerstrider.com).
- Keenfit's video is on the company's Web site (www.keenfit.com).
- Komperdell's video is currently available only in Europe.
- LEKI includes a DVD, free with each set of poles.
- PoleAbout has a basic instructional video on its Web site (www.poleabout.com).
- SkiWalking includes an instructional DVD, free with every set of poles.

Besides the product-related DVDs above, *Nordic Walking— The Ultimate Fitness Experience* is a 40-minute instructional DVD put out by zFit.com, a company run by trainer Bernd Zimmermann, who also founded and is president of the American Nordic Walking Association.

is a function of time and speed, pay attention initially to how long you are walking. If you use a pedometer, that instrument can translate your steps into distance to give you a good idea of how far you are walking. If you are a beginner, don't be too hard on yourself. Keep in mind that the athlete's starting point could well be (or exceed) the new exerciser's goals. LEKI poles come with an informational hangtag that includes some tips—hints, not pole tips—to help you set reasonable goals.

Two companies have identified levels of fitness and accomplishment. LEKI has parsed Nordic Walking into three levels of fitness and suggested a three-step workout for each. I've paraphrased LEKI's levels slightly without altering their meaning. Use them as guidelines, not gospel. They are:

Beginner/Occasional Walker
1. 5-minute warmup.
2. 15- to 30-minute easy walk with poles, pushing off slightly to create resistance and work the upper body. LEKI says that you will feel it in your chest, back and arms.
3. 5-minute cool-down, walking at a very easy pace, and then stretching.

Intermediate/Walk Three or More Days Per Week
1. 5-minute warmup.
2. 30- to 60-minute brisk walk with poles, pushing off more aggressively to create more resistance and work and strengthen the upper body. LEKI suggests that this is time to begin working on your rhythm.
3. 5-minute cool-down, walking at an easy pace, and then stretching.

Conditioned Athlete
1. 5-minute warm up.
2. 60-plus-minute walk with poles, emphasizing a swifter, stronger endurance stride and pace, including hill climbs, walking against the wind, interval training or such strength exercises as lunges incorporated into the walk.
3. 10-minute cool-down, gradually reducing the walking pace and intensity, and then stretching.

Fittrek developed seven different variants on basic Nordic Walking technique for different terrain applications (see Seven from Fittrek on page 127) and also came up with its Linear Progression of Intensity to help Nordic Walkers gauge their intensity and progress. In the Fittrek lexicon, you will therefore find basic technique, fast walking, off-road and on-road variations, and uphill and downhill technique.

Regardless of which progression you learn from, know that the benefits are significant, but don't get carried away in the expectation department. When you read that walking with poles can burn up to 45% more calories than covering the same distance at the same speed without poles, that refers to the conditioned athlete, working hard, not the occasional or even intermediate Nordic Walker. But most important for beginners is that everyone has to start somewhere, and for a person who has not been exercising, LEKI's beginner/occasional or Fittrek's basic Nordic Walker guidelines are a very good start.

The bottom line for new Nordic Walkers is to get out and do it. You will probably want to increase your speed, distance and intensity as you gain experience, but you have to begin laying a Nordic Walking foundation before you build on it.

Laughing All the Way

New Nordic Walkers are often self-conscious about going out with walking poles and being the butt of such comments as, "Don't you know there's no snow?" If someone calls that to you, you can joke back, "I know. I'm going out looking for it," or "If you find any, let me know." Or you can just smile—perhaps smugly—knowing that while Nordic Walking might look odd to the uninitiated, you are doing yourself and your health a world of good.

Instructor and enthusiast Marek Zalewski tends to use such one-liners directed at him as an opportunity to enlighten others to the benefits of Nordic Walking by responding with something to the effect of, "I suppose that you are familiar with the use of poles only with skis. Haven't you heard of trekking and hiking poles and of Nordic Walking poles? Well, these happen to be Nordic Walking poles. I could show you how you could get in really great shape with their help and maybe even lose that sagging belly, but I 've really got better things to do right now. Have a great day!"

Besides, how many of us really care what a wise-cracking stranger might say in passing?

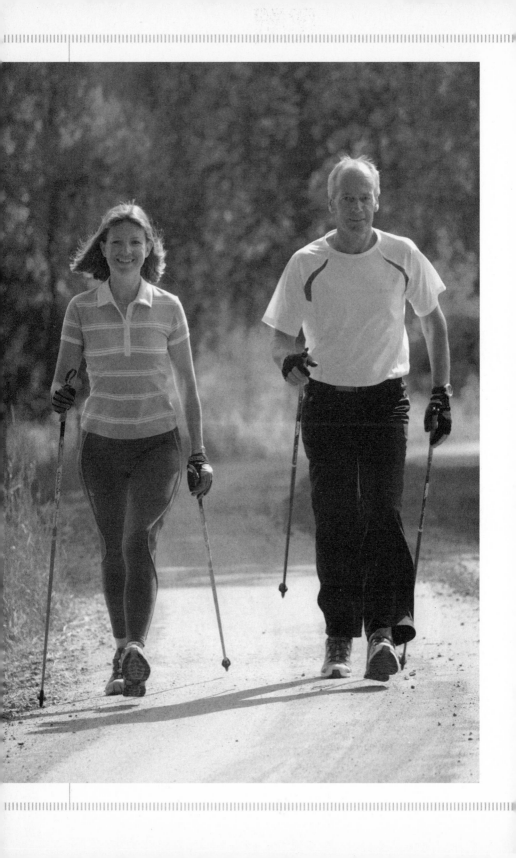

6

Something
Extra

Arguably the most remarkable aspect of Nordic Walking is its extreme versatility. It fits an astonishingly wide range of needs, physical abilities and desires in people of all ages and physical condition. It can be done virtually anywhere—in urban, suburban and rural settings, in mountainous regions, along the seashore and on the plains. And it can be done in all but the most extreme kinds of weather, and when snow covers the ground, snowshoeing or cross-country skiing is a great winter substitute.

GO WITH A GROUP

Solo walks can be contemplative and certainly are good exercise, but walking with others carries both social and motivational benefits—and in some areas, there is safety in numbers for those with such concerns. For everyone, however, no matter where he or she lives or travels, Nordic Walking is an ideal group activity. Remember the surprising and satisfying characteristic of its "rate of perceived exertion," meaning that you will actually be working harder aerobically than you feel. For a fuller explanation, see "Getting to the Heart of the Matter" in Chapter 1, page 3. In practical terms, that translates to the ability to Nordic Walk and carry on a conversation with your walking partners without shouting or getting out of breath.

A group can offer something for all levels of Nordic Walkers and all personalities—for natural leaders and content followers, for those who like to lean on someone and those who like to be depended upon, for trailblazers and those who are not comfortable in new situations. Nordic Walking with others also means that you'll have buddies to encourage you if you are having a draggy day and are falling behind your usual pace, and that you'll be able to do the same for others when they are down. Experienced Nordic Walkers are generally willing to share little tips with newbies—not instruction per se, but encouragement and perhaps a bit of advice now and again.

By its very nature, a group will set a tempo that helps pull new Nordic Walkers along. Those who are naturally fast seem to like setting the pace and do so automatically, while those who prefer to walk at a more restrained speed ramp up their energy. Don't think of group walks like military units or marching bands. Each participant will eventually go at his or her own pace, but that pace might be slower or faster than going it alone.

Recognizing that opportunities exist for trained Nordic Walking guides who prefer not to go for real instructor certification, the American Nordic Walking Association organizes Nordic Walking Guide workshops, and LEKI similarly has developed its Community Walk Leader program. The same master coaches who conduct the Certification Seminars give ANWA's 3-hour guide workshops. Neither program requires previous teaching experience or even a Nordic Walking background, and both including techniques and tools for safely and effectively introducing family, friends and colleagues to Nordic Walking—a further testimonial to how simple Nordic Walking really is.

Finding an established Nordic Walking group does still present something of a challenge. You can, of course, take an ANWA, Exerstrider, INWA, LEKI or other workshop, and then get together with classmates, start your own group or find an existing one in your community. Some instructors form groups from previous students. Often people who get along well in a class agree to meet regularly to go for Nordic Walks—with or without their instructor. Planned communities, with organized recreation programs or local hospital wellness programs, especially those geared to retirees, are increasingly adding Nordic Walking to their schedules. A handful of dedicated Nordic Walking clubs have been formed in this country, with the Association of Nordic Walking Clubs established as a clearinghouse for information. To date, the information is minimal, but that might change over time. The clubs in that association are concentrated in Florida. At this writing, the association which appears to be loosely connected with Fittrek, is not particularly active, but perhaps it eventually will be. Some running stores, running clubs and Volkssport-type walking clubs have Nordic Walking groups—and as the sport catches on they will be ever more inclined to do so. If you can't find a local group, request one—or start one.

If you want to Nordic Walk for a good cause, register for any of the numerous pledge walks around the calendar and around the country, and ask whether poles are permitted. Organizers are generally hospitable to Nordic Walkers, just as many are to participants pushing baby carriages and strollers. These not-for-profit organizations are primarily interested in raising money through donations and/or pledges and less paranoid than race organizers about the hazards that poles might potentially present. When people begin showing up at these fundraisers with poles and nothing harmful occurs, it will most likely go a long way toward making Nordic Walking an accepted part of races and other mass events.

North American Volkssport Associations

Volkssport is German for "peoples' sport." Swimming, cycling and, most of all, walking are activities encompassed in the Volkssport concept, and of these, no activity is more universal than walking. In North America, the related word Volksmarch means a non-competitive 6-mile (10-kilometer) walk—neither a pledge walk nor a race, but rather a fun activity to do with a group, with family, friends, a pet or alone—and also some shorter walks. Literally thousands of Volkssport clubs around the world are allied with each other through the International Volkssport Federation (IVV). The American Volkssport Association includes 350 walking clubs and more than 3,000 guided walking events annually in all 50 states. Some 44 individual clubs, two provincial associations and several affiliate entities belong to the Canadian Volkssport Federation (CVF)—La Fédération Canadienne Volkssport (FCV) to Francophone Canadians. All organized Volkssport events are open to anyone who wishes to participate and are free or low-cost (generally under $7).

The AVA's and CVF's Web sites are goldmines for walking information, with events listed by state or province, date and other information, most important a contact person who can answer questions about the use of poles. There are also suggestions for marked and/or mapped trails for those who take non-group walks. These are rated from 1 to 5, ranging from a paved or well-maintained trail without significant hills to a very difficult walk over rough fields or woods, including steep hills, high elevations trails, very rough and/or uneven terrain, and steep or unstable inclines. Like Nordic Walking itself, trails identified by the AVA are suitable for all levels of interest and conditioning. People who like to keep track of their walking activities like the rewards and recognition for the distance they've put in or other goals they have achieved in Volkssport-sanctioned walks—for example, walking in all 50 states or all 50 state capitals, accomplishing 10 walks along Great Lakes shores, completing 20 walking routes on named islands along coastlines of rivers or lakes, and so on.

You do not even have to leave home to be a member of an interesting group—a virtual Nordic Walking eCommunity that meets in cyberspace. Author and Nordic Walking instructor David Downer established a forum in January 2006 and continues to moderate—now with co-moderators in several countries. To sign up (free), go to www.nordicwalkingecommunity.com and follow the directions. Once you have registered, you will discover an ongoing Nordic Walking conversation, mostly about technique, instruction, poles and footwear, but also touching on clothing, group Nordic Walks, competitive Nordic Walking and places to walk. Many people on the list are in Britain, where David Downer lives, but the shared ideas and conversations on most topics are universal and make the forum feel like a real community—albeit one without walls or borders.

REHAB FROM INJURY OR SURGERY

By taking stress from the lower body, Nordic Walking poles are well suited to rehabilitation from ankle, knee and hip injuries or even joint-replacement surgery. Some physical therapists and physicians find them useful for patients transitioning from crutches to walking unaided. Like crutches, poles are bilateral (meaning the user has two of them and is supposed to use them evenly on both sides) but restrict movement. By contrast, canes are unilateral (one side) and provide some support and stability, but can make the user feel lop-sided. Some medical practitioners work with patients following cardiac bypass surgery with

Nordic Walking as well after the surgical site has healed and they are satisfied with heart function as shown by monitored treadmill walks. Stroke victims have also reported success in regaining function with Nordic Walking. None of these conditions call for self-diagnosed Nordic Walking, but rather a program worked out in conjunction with a doctor and a trained and open-minded rehabilitation therapist.

DOG WALKING

Nordic Walking and dog walking are not incompatible, unless the dog cannot be trained to stay out of the way of poles. See "Doggone Clever Leash Systems" on page 95 for leash systems that attach to the waist (the walker's, not the dog's).

NORDIC WALKING IN UNIFORM

The stereotypical soldier is able to run for miles carrying a rifle and a heavy pack on his or her back, do fast push-ups by the score, march in formation and do a snappy salute when required, no matter how tired he or she is. The military now has discovered Nordic Walking as an enjoyable way to stay in shape and keep a competitive edge. Much of the credit goes to Sue Bozgoz, a U.S. Army Lieutenant Colonel (retired) and an ALL Army Marathoner and Track Runner who has coached more than 10,000 walkers, runners and Nordic Walkers and has completed more than 51 marathons, including the annual U.S. Marine Corps Marathon. In 2007, the Army kicked off its 232nd birthday celebration with 5K and 10K foot races and, astonishingly, the first-ever 5K Nordic Pole Walking Championships at Fort McPherson, GA. "The activity [Nordic Walking] is not only excellent for the elite athletes, it is a great workout for everyone at all levels of fitness, especially soldiers who put stress on their tendons, ligaments and muscles everyday while training in combat boots," said Bozgoz, assistant race director, who also consults with Foot Solutions, a chain of footwear retail stores committed to promoting Nordic Walking and involved with these military races.

Some schools run by the Department of Defense for military dependents on European bases have begun incorporating Nordic Walking and other wellness activities into their physical education programs.

PUSHING THE NORDIC WALKING ENVELOPE

This book is not intended as a high-athletic-level training guide, but knowing a bit about options for advanced Nordic Walkers who wish to leap to the next level with more energetic forms of the sport. Detailed information on interval training, aerobic versus anaerobic exercise, ideal training schedules and other regimens undertaken by serious athletes can be applied to Nordic Walking as well, but remain beyond the ambitions of this book.

- Skipping is a schoolyard movement that with the addition of poles is lighthearted, fun and energetic. Children particularly enjoy Nordic skipping, but so do fit grownups who are kids at heart. Jogging or running with poles adds to the workout. Jogging and running use the entire foot rather than the heel-to-toe rolling motion of walking, and also permits both feet to be off the ground, briefly, at the same time. Especially when running, the stride will be even longer than the most aggressive walking.

- Bounding or hill bounding is an intense activity derived directly from the cross-country skiing dry-land training techniques that spawned Nordic Walking. It is essentially running up and down hills with big aggressive strides. Even well-conditioned athletes can quickly raise their heart rates with a short ski-bounding interval. Similarly, plyometrics with poles provide a dynamite strength- and power-building workout for high-level athletic training. With arms outstretched and poles planted firmly on each side, leap explosively from side to side, providing a plyometric movement sequence with poles.

- In-line skating, which was very hot in the late 1980s through the mid- to late '90s, has cooled off considerably in the United States, but popularity issues notwithstanding, hard-core enthusiasts who want to add an upper-body component to their skating pick up long poles and combine the two activities. The technique is similar to the skating version of cross-country skiing. It requires some adjustment, because you have to make sure that the skates and poles don't get tangled during the sideways push-off—and if you are "Nordic skating" on a congested path or one with bushes and trees growing close to the pavement, you must be especially mindful as you speed along with flying poles.

Nordic Walkers who want something extra might be tempted to add ankle weights or wrist weights, but many experts caution that these put too much stress on the joints during an intense activity that already burdens the joints, especially the knees but also the hips and ankles. Fittrek offers resistance bands that can be used to increase the workload, and Gymstick poles are designed with built-in resistance coils to incorporate strength-training into every walk (see Chapter 2). Some aggressive Nordic Walkers wear weighted vests to ratchet up the workout, but others just recommend doing lots of up- and downhill work, maintaining the flat-ground pace—if the route actually has hills. As indicated earlier, Fittrek's technique is, at this writing, the only Nordic Walking program recognized by ACE (American Council on Exercise), AFFA (Aerobics and Fitness Federation of America) and Canadian Fitness Professionals (Can Fit Pro) and pioneered the training of club-affiliated fitness professionals to become Nordic Walking instructors.

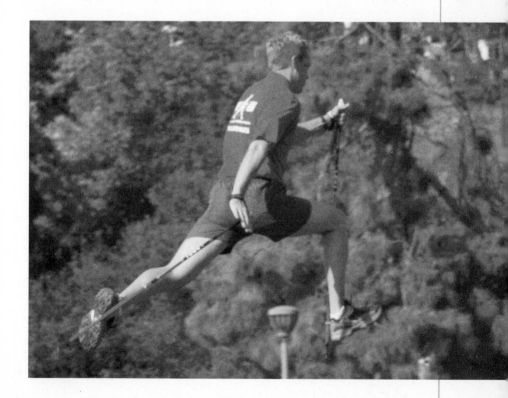

Ed Urbanski on Regaining Fitness Through Nordic Walking

Ed, now a multiply trained and certified Nordic Walking instructor, got into the sport in its earliest days, when the equipment choices were extremely limited and Nordic Walking didn't really have a name. As a cross-country ski racer back in the 1970s, he used his ski poles for "hill bounding," an aggressive training technique that involved running up hills in summer using poles to push up during the ascent. He also used poles for roller skiing, another summer training option. He kept going hard until, like so many serious athletes, he began paying the price for years of training and running. With no cartilage left in his knees, those joints gave out. After joint replacement surgery on both knees, he recommenced walking with poles. This energetic resident of Greendale, WI, is both an ANWA and an Exerstride Method certified instructor:

"I began pole walking in 1988, when I bought my first set of Exerstriders from Tom Rutlin. I used them for several years, but then set them aside. I completed the Hawaiian Ironman World Championship in 1987 at age 50, but after I stopped my aerobic exercises and started power lifting, my weight slowly went from a 'lean' 175 to a 'fat' 255. By age 60, I was on the verge of becoming a type 2 diabetic. Finally I decided that I didn't want to live the rest of my life as a fat man. Then, in 2004, I had my knees replaced and the next year, I began Exerstriding or Nordic Walking again. Now [in 2007] at age 70, my current weight is 205 pounds, with my goal of 190 in sight, and I am no longer considered to be pre-diabetic. I still have and use that first set of poles, particularly in the wintertime. Exerstriders do not have straps, but rather have a unique, ergonomic grip that works very well without straps. Wisconsin winters get very cold, and I like to wear heavy mittens when I walk, and therefore Exerstriders work very well. My wife, who does not like straps on her poles, also uses Exerstrider poles. I like Exerstriders and also consider LEKI to be the best poles with straps. I became one of the first Leki instructors in March 2006 and an advanced level ANWA certified instructor in May 2007, and I received my certified Exerstride Method Nordic Walking instructor certificate on September 2007. Best part is that I get to teach others an activity that I truly believe in and enjoy."

COMPETITION

While Nordic Walking is primarily for fitness and fun, some competitive souls like to race, either recreationally or seriously. Some races simply prohibit the use of poles. Others permit Nordic Walking but with certain restrictions—perhaps requiring Nordic Walkers to refrain from using poles at the start, the finish and/or a congested part of the course. Still other race organizers tolerate Nordic Walkers, while some now truly welcome them. Canadian organizers have been more open to poles than their U.S. counterparts. In any event, Nordic Walkers are often grouped into walking divisions along with participants who compete without poles. An increasing number of serious Nordic Walkers—notably competitive runners whose knees have been giving them problems—are champing at the bit for more Nordic Walking competitions, and there is considerable debate in the British Nordic Walking community as to whether races open only to pole walkers are better for the sport or whether exposing pole-less competitors to it will benefit its growth.

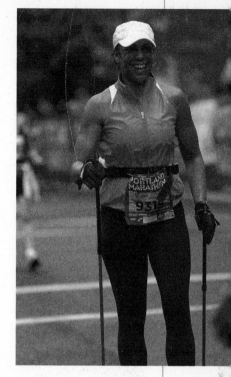

The Portland (Oregon) Marathon deserves special mention. It was the first major U.S. distance race to include a separate Nordic Walking category. Since 2005 it also has served as the Nordic Walking World Championship at the regulation marathon distance and more recently also at the 5K distance. Fittrek, which initially sponsored this championship component, created guidelines available to race directors—not just for marathons, but also applicable for road races of various lengths—on how to integrate Nordic Walking safely into a foot-race. These were supplanted in 2008 by new "protocols" guiding Nordic Walkers in footraces (see page 151 for the entire document).

The most common distances for Nordic Walking divisions of foot races, whether seriously competitive or purely recreational, are 5K, 10K and half-marathon (13.1 miles), plus the occasional full marathon. Some race organizers restrict the distances for Nordic Walking, while others impose a time limit for completion of the full distance for all participants. Nordic Walking coaches and running stores with group training programs that are located in areas with competitions that permit poles often offer special sessions for Nordic Walkers.

Other North American races that permit participants to use poles include the Denver Marathon; Mayor's Marathon in Anchorage; San Diego Marathon; Lake Tahoe Marathon, California; Indy Classic Marathon, Indianapolis; Woolly Mammoth Classic/Hulda Hilfiker Memorial Run/Walk, Brill, Wisconsin; and Sunrise Stampede in Longmont, Colorado. In Canada, Nordic Walkers are welcome in the Sun Run in Vancouver, the Vancouver Marathon, the Vancouver Island Marathon and the Edge to Edge Marathon, (also on Vancouver Island on Canada's West Coast) and the Marathon by the Sea, St. John, New Brunswick in the East.

Numerous walk/run fund raisers for good causes are held all over the country, and they are generally pole-friendly. As Nordic Walking grows in popularity, other races will permit and eventually encourage it.

In 2007, Fittrek's Dan Barrett and Dr. Tony Weaver of the Association of Nordic Walking Clubs came up with training guidelines to help prepare for the grueling marathon distance. They recommend that training begin for individuals who have been Nordic Walking for at least 6 months to 1 year before the event and that they already have a base of walking four times a week, averaging at least 15 miles (or better, 20 to 25) a week. From this, they developed a day-by-day 19-week training schedule. While Fittrek no longer sponsors the Nordic Walking part of the Portland Marathon, the training schedule is still available on-line at portlandmarathon.org/images/nordictrainingguide.pdf.

Across the Atlantic, both on the Continent and in Great Britain, races abound either that permit, encourage or are focused on Nordic Walking. For example, the four events of England's Lakeland Trails Series include both Nordic Walking-only and mixed events. Sweden's three-day Lidingöloppet takes place near Stockholm and includes the Lidingö Stavgång, a Nordic Walking-only event along a beautiful 10K course with a shorter 4K option. The Berlin Marathon welcomes Nordic Walkers, and in the southern part of the country, the Allgäuer Nordic Walking Marathon in Ottobeuern is not burdened with accommodating Nordic Walkers in a generally pole-free race, but is exclusively for competitors with poles. Intriguingly, the course is

Nordic Walking Competition Protocol

In 2008, Portland Marathon organizers adopted the protocol below that was written by Malcolm Jarvis and David Downer of www.NordicWalkingeCommunity.com with input from both sides of the Atlantic.

The Nordic Walking Protocol is constructed in two parts: Safety Rules/ Nordic Walking Etiquette and Guiding Principles.

Criteria concerning safety are given the status of rules, as safe walking must have primacy. However, how a participant walks, and the technique he or she adopts is a matter of personal choice, and this is intentionally left open. The underlying ethos of these principles is to be inclusive and they are therefore designed to allow any form of "fitness-walking with purpose made poles."

Safety Rules and Nordic Walking Etiquette

1. Show consideration to your fellow participants and act as ambassadors for Nordic Walking.
2. Nordic Walkers are asked to avoid walking in groups in such a way that might impede the progress of others. A faster participant who wishes to overtake is requested to give polite audible warning by saying "passing on the right (or left) please".
3. Where the event is road based, walking poles should have purpose made rubber "asphalt paws" attached throughout and participants should carry a spare pair. This is designed to prevent potential injury, aid traction and reduce noise.
4. Please remember to keep your poles pointing downwards at all times, except when changing paws.
5. Except in an emergency, please do not lay your poles on the ground during the event.
6. If there is a need to adjust poles, or replace asphalt paws, move to the side of the course, and take great care when working on your poles.
7. When taking fluids, or food, or for personal attendance, by all means free one pole but carry it close to the body.

laid out as a 10.5-kilometer circuit with event distances a multiple of that distance, which is roughly 6 miles. The eight distances centered around the Swissalpine Marathon are run on trails in the magnificent Swiss Alps around Davos. One component is the 21K (around 13-mile) Nordic Walk.

Guiding principles

1. **Walking**—This special event category is primarily a walking category, so each participant must maintain one foot in contact with the ground throughout, in order to prevent being able to jog or run.
2. **Walking**—As a walking event this category does not envisage the use of roller blades, (as in Nordic Blading) nor any other kind of assistance device.
3. **Poles**—Participants are expected to use two poles actively and continuously throughout the event, except when taking fluids or food, or during personal attendance, or in an emergency.
4. **Poles**—In order to allow the adoption of any form of pole walking technique, poles can either have demi gloves (straps) or be strapless. Poles can be of any type or manufacture provided they are suited to the purpose, i.e. being designed for fitness-walking, and they may be of one piece or adjustable design.
5. **Technique**—There is but one simple requirement: the participant is asked to adopt a Nordic Walking style where the pole tips are planted somewhere behind a line extending from the leading hand plumb to the ground. Apart from this, there is NO control over the style actually adopted—we call upon your sense of fairness and personal integrity!

Judith Yaaqoubi on Nordic Walking Rather Than Running a Marathon

After this Edmonds, Washington, resident competed in the Portland Marathon, she was transformed from a runner to a Nordic Walker. Here is her report:

"I trained the first 9 months of 2006 to run a half-marathon in Washington but hurt my knee in September. I was so frustrated that I could not keep on training and most likely could not do the marathon. After a couple of weeks of doing nothing, I remembered the Nordic Walking instruction I had on my vacations in Germany (I amGerman, and it seems that everybody there 'does it'). I started theNordic Walking, and my knee did not hurt a bit. Lucky me that I bought a pair of no-brand poles in Germany during my last vacation. I did not find new ones here so far.

"Still frustrated that I could not do my half-marathon, I looked into half marathons that allowed Nordic Walking. I e-mailed the organizer of one marathon and was told that they were worried that people would get hurt with my poles. It was then, that I found the information about the Portland Marathon on the Monday before the race and signed up immediately. It was a full marathon, but I was confident that my running training would get me through it. The day before the marathon I met Dan [Barrett] from Fittrek, who gave me some new paws for my poles—which was really necessary. Dan is the official sponsor of the Nordic Walking part of the Portland Marathon, the only marathon to my knowledge in the northwest part of the U.S.A. at least, that allows officially for Nordic Walking (and has its own championship).

"The morning of the race, we met at the very end of the field. We were about 18 Nordic Walkers and were told the day before to start at the very end. Again, also in Portland, they seemingly were a little worried about what we do with the poles and who we [might] hurt. In my opinion, it does not make very much sense to let Nordic Walkers start at the end of the field. The risk of hurting other people is definitely higher if you have to get through a dense field of slower walkers than if you start in your own pace field. But, obviously, nobody was hurt or knocked over with the poles.

"Again, we were about 18 Nordic Walkers (among 5,000 runners/walkers!). The race itself was very well organized: 36 bands along the way, every mile or so water and nutrition bars and lots of people to cheer us on. I forgot to mention that this was my first marathon... I am not familiar with how it works in different cities. We Nordic Walkers split up fairly soon as everybody followed their own pace. The first 10 miles were great for me. I was highly motivated. The weather was perfect—not too sunny, a little cloudy. I just followed the clicks of my poles and paid attention to my technique. Nobody controlled the stroke or stride. I think there are too many different techniques out there to validate just one.

"At mile 13, it got a little more difficult as the course followed a pretty industrial part of the city, no more bands for about 3 or 4 miles. I then realized that I did not have the right shoes for Nordic Walking. I was walking in my running shoes as I did not want to risk blisters in new walking shoes, but I got them anyway after 5 miles. By mile 13, my shinbones started to hurt badly It seems that my running shoes had elevated heels that put some extra stress on my shins. I pushed through the pain. At about mile 15, my body started hurting. My shoulders and arms got kind of numb, because I did not train for Nordic Walking and, obviously, when running, you do not use a lot of the muscle groups you do for Nordic Walking.

"But the excitement of getting to the end made me finish the marathon. I finished in 6 hours and 18 minutes. My goal was to stay under 6 hours. So not too bad, I think. The Nordic Walking winner finished in 5 hours and a little bit. I, personally, am now completely hooked on Nordic Walking. I just finished my instructor training and am working on spreading the word in Seattle."

Author's note: In 2007, the Portland Marathon actually recorded nearly 8,000 finishers. Also, Dan Barrett and Fittrek were involved in sponsorship when Yaaqoubi entered in 2007 but that is no longer the case.

TAKE OFF ON A WALKING VACATION

Nordic Walking can take you around the block or around the world. Ironically, walking vacations are more difficult to find close to home in the U.S. than abroad. Unlike Europe, where regular, organized Nordic Walking opportunities abound at mountain, lake and beach resorts from the Alps to the Algarve to the Arctic Circle, only a select few North American destinations have committed to offering programs with the availability of poles and basic instruction. Most of these are ski or mountain resorts that offer it during the off-season (i.e., summer). Colorado's Beaver Creek Hiking Center at the Beaver Creek ticket office in the center of the village was one of the first to commit to Nordic Walking as well as offering guided hiking tours. The hiking center organizes 90-minute group Nordic Walks at 10:00 a.m. daily, including the use of LEKI poles and a water bottle. Call 970-845-9090 for more information or to confirm that the meeting time and place have not changed. The Sports and Wellness Center at Stoweflake, a resort in Stowe, VT, includes Nordic Walking as one of its summer activity options. Stoweflake can be reached by calling 800-253-2232 or 802-253-7355. Quebec-based Chinook adventure merits singling out for its corps of Nordic Walking instructors in 15 cities, for organizing a Nordic Walking festival and for Nordic Walking trips in Canada and elsewhere; contact 888-599-0999 or go to www.chinookadventure. com.

Wellness weeks or weekends increasingly include Nordic Walking as one of the activities. Some places occasionally scheduled Nordic Walking programs, but their continuation has depended as much on the availability of a trained instructor as on the demand from guests. Places that schedule guided hiking programs, nature walks and family walks would seem to be fertile fields for sowing the Nordic Walking seed. If you are already a Nordic Walker and have your own poles, or find a nearby sporting goods shop that carries them, you can join a walking group and make it into a Nordic Walk for yourself. Nature walks and family walks do not really lend themselves to energetic walking with poles, but hiking and adult walking programs often do. You need to be resourceful and ask.

Assembling an independent Nordic Walking vacation is fairly straightforward. In the countryside of Europe and the British Isles, well-marked walking paths and trekking trails abound. Local tourist offices provide maps and can also advise you about groups that you can join or the numerous walking festivals that visitors can also take part in. When walking on the Continent or in the British Isles, you can either do a loop or follow a route to a nearby village and catch a train, bus or taxi back to the place you are staying. In addition to seeing splendid scenery at a step-by-step pace, this is really a wonderful way to meet Europeans or Brits.

Dedicated Nordic Walking trips are still rare, but multi-day walking tours in North America. Europe, New Zealand, Asia and Latin America are getting more popular every year. Participants generally move along at their own pace, often with a lead and a tail guide so that no one in the middle gets lost. Luggage transport and meals are normally included, which means that guests can concentrate on the scenery and the joy of walking. There is no reason you can't take your poles and invoke Nordic Walking technique. Some itineraries are tailored for seniors (over 50 or 55 or 60), others for families and still others only for women. Some are luxurious, while others are simpler.

Among the other U.S. and Canadian travel providers known for their walking programs are:

- Abercromie & Kent, 800-554-7016, www.abercombiekent.com
- Austin-Lehman Adventures, 800-575-2540,
  www.austinlehman.com
- Backroads, 800-462-2848, www.backroads.com
- Classic Journeys, 800-200-3887, 858-454-5004,
  www.classicjourneys.com
- Country Walkers, 800-464-9255, www.countrywalkers.com
- Cross Country International Walking Vacations, 800-828-8768,
  www.walkingvacations.com
- Elderhostel, 800-454-5768, www.elderhostel.org
- European Walking Tours (Swiss company with a U.S. office),
  217-398-0058, 800-231-8448, www.walkingtours.com
- Experience Plus, 800-685-4565, www.experienceplus.com
- Euro-Bike & Walking Tours, 800-321-6060, 815-758-8851,
  www.eurobike.com
- New England Hiking Holidays, 800-869-0949,
  www.nehikingholidays.com
- Ramblers 800-724-8801, 703-680-4276, www.ramblers.com

- The Walking Connection, 800-295-WALK, www.walkingconnection.com
- Walking Softly Adventures, 888-743-0723, www.walkingsoftly.com
- The Wayfarers, 800-249-4620, 401-849-5087, www.thewayfarers. com
- Trips & Trails, 800-581-HIKE, www.tahoetrips.com
- Van Gogh Tours 802-767-3457, 800-435-6192, www.vangoghtours.com

Savvy North Americans can also plug into British tour operators' itineraries like those offered by Ramblers International (+44 (0) 1707 331133, www.ramblersholidays.co.uk), Footloose (a U.K. company with a U.S. number, 800-221-0596, www.footloose.com); HF Holidays (+44 (0) 20 8732 1220, www.hfholidays.co.uk) and Moving Feet (+44 (0) 7809 264 939, www.movingfeet.co.uk). An on-line resource with links to walking, hiking and trekking tours is www.WebWalking.com.

Millions of North Americans take cruises every year. Cruise ships are popular for their abundant food served practically around the clock. To help passengers work off some of those calories and make room for more food, most large ships have some kind of a promenade deck with a non-slip surface and distance markers to keep track of how far people have jogged or walked. If you are preparing for a cruise, slip a pair of poles with rubber paws affixed into one of your bags and take advantage of the obstacle-free outdoor deck. If anyone questions your equipment, show them the poles and point out that ships welcome passengers with crutches, canes or wheelchairs, so your poles should present no problem.

Bon voyage. Or rather bon "walkage."

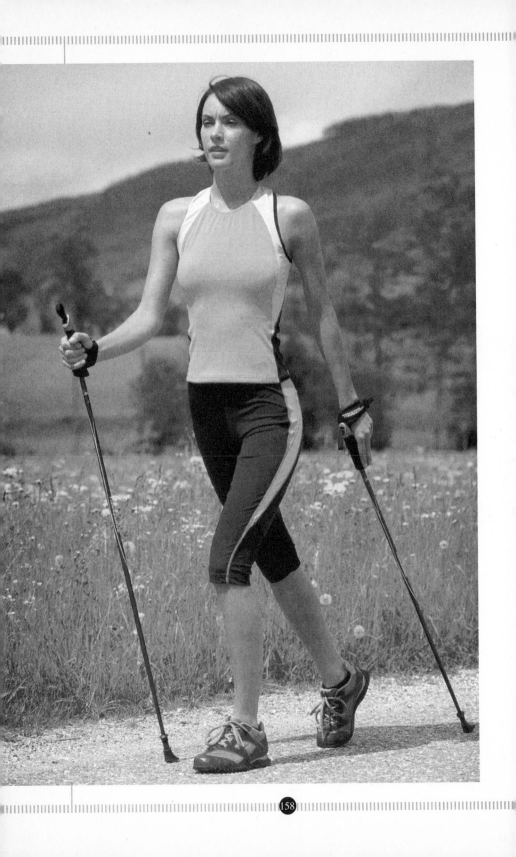

RESOURCES

ORGANIZATIONS

American Nordic Walking Association (ANWA)
P.O. Box 491205
Los Angeles, CA 90049
323-244-2519
www.anwa.us

American Volkssport Association (AVA)
1001 Pat Booker Road, Suite 101
Universal City, TX 78148
210-659-2112
www.ava.org

Asociación Mexicana de Caminata Nordica
No street or mailing address or city available
(+52 55) 56 31 26 00
www.caminatanordica.com.mx

Association of Nordic Walking Clubs (ANWC)
No street address, post office box or zip code available
Miami Beach, FL
800-345-1004 or 305-785-6289
www.nordicwalkingclubs.com

Australasian Nordic Walking Association (ANWA)
P.O. Box 450
Kaiapoi 7962, New Zealand
(+64) 03 375 5062
www.anwa.org.nz

Canadian Nordic Walking Association (CNWA)
78 Skipton Trail
Aurora, ON L4G 7P7
905-713-6164
www.cnwa.info

Canadian Nordic Fitness
306 - 15468 Roper Ave.
White Rock, BC V4B 2G5
www.canadiannordicfitness.com

Canadian Volkssport Federation (CVA)
P.O. Box 2668
Station "D"
Ottawa, ON K1P 5W7
613-234-7333
www.walks.ca

International Nordic Walking Federation (INWA)
Herculesstraat 14
1973 VP IJmuiden
The Netherlands
(+31) 640 518 445
www.inwa-nordicwalking.com
The INWF Web site also has links to member organizations that at
this writing include Australia, Andorra, Austria, Belgium, China,
Croatia, Denmark, Estonia, Finland, Germany, Great Britain,
Hungary, Ireland, Italy, Japan, Latvia, Luxembourg, Netherlands,
New Zealand, Norway, Poland, Slovenia, South Korea, Spain,
Sweden, Switzerland and the United States.

International Nordic Fitness Organisation (INFO)
www.nordicfitness.dnv-online.de
Umbrella organization for several promotional and certifying
entities including:
- Asociación de Nordic Walking de España (Spain),
  www.nordicwalking-ane.es (Web site in Spanish)
- Deutscher Nordic Walking/Deutscher Inline Verband (Germany,
  Austria), www.dnv-online.de (Web site in German)
- Associazione Nordic Fitness Italiana (ANI, Italy),
  www.nordicwalking.it (Web site in Italian and German)
- Swiss Nordic Fitness Organisation, www.swissnordicfitness.info
  (Web site in German)

Nordic Walking Union e.V.
Rathenaustraße 10
67547 Worms, Germany
(+49) 0 62 41 / 305 693
www.nwunion.de

Nordic Walking USA (INWA affiliate)
2629 Main Street #700
Santa Monica, CA 90405
310-399-8522
www.nordicbody.com

Scottish Nordic Walking Association
No address or phone number
www.scottishnordicwalkingassociation.co.uk/

POLES

**Alpina Sports Corporation
(importer of Exel and Masters poles)**
P.O. Box 23
Hanover, NH 03755
800-425-7462 or
603-448-3101
www.alpinasports.com

Balanced GmbH
Ob der Kirche 7
7306 Fläsch, Switzerland
(+41) 81 330 19 39
www.balanced.ch

Boomyah International LLC
1003 South Emerson Street, Suite 100
Denver, CO 80209
303-765-4615
www.boomyah.com

Buddy System
c/o Chicks In Charge, LLC
3412 Lake Vanessa Cr NW
Salem, OR 97304
888-363-2818 or 503-363-3135
www.buddysys.com

Exel USA, Inc.
See Alpina Sports
www.alpinesports.com

Exerstrider Products, Inc.,
P.O. Box 3087
Madison, WI 53704-0087
608-223-9321
www.exerstrider.com

Fischer Sports U.S.A.
60 Dartmouth Drive
Auburn, NH 03032
603-314-7110
http://us.fischer-ski.com/en/
or
Fischer GmbH
Fischerstraße 8
A-4910 Ried im Innkreis, Austria
(+43) 7752 909 0
www.fischer-skis.com

Fittrek
535 29th Street
Miami Beach, FL 33140
800-345-1004 or 305-751-3800
www.fittrek.com

Gabel Sports Group North America
2573 des Tulipes
Vaudreuil QC J7V 9K8, Canada
450-455-1414
www.gabel-sport.com

Gymstick
Gymstick International
5406 Mollys Glen
Mineral, VA 23117
800-788-9143
www.gymstick.net

Iwalk2
c/o Canadian Nordic Walking Association
78 Skipton Trail
Aurora, ON L4G 7P7
903-713-6164
www.cnwa.info

Joy
See Balanced GmbH

Kahtoola, Inc.
450 River Run Road
Flagstaff, AZ 86001
866-330-8030
www.kahtoola.com

Keenfit
2684 Casa Loma Road
Kelowna B.C. V1Z 1T5
Canada
250-769-9241 or 877-KEEN-FIT (533-6348)
www.keenfit.com

Komperdell Sportartikel Ges.m.b.H.
Wagnermühle 30
A-5310 Mondsee, Austria
(+43) 6232 4201 0
www.komperdell.com

LEKI USA
458 Sonwil Drive
Buffalo, NY 14225
www.leki.com
or
LEKI Lenhart GmbH
Karl-Arnold Strasse 30
D-73230 Kirchheim /Teck, Germany
www.leki.de

Masters SRL
c/o Alpina Sports
93 Etna Road
P.O. Box 23
Hanover, NH 03755
800-425-7462 or 603-448-3101
or
Via Capitelvecchio, 29
36061 Bassano del Grappa (VI), Italy
(+39) 0424 524133 r.a.
www.masters.it

Nordixx
c/o NordicPoleWalkingUSA LLC
P.O. BOX 2162
Naples, FL 34102-2162
239-298-2612
www.nordicpolewalkingusa.com

PAD-CENTRE
Kunderi 37-5
10121 Tallinn, Estonia
(+372) 0 60 26 295
www.poleabout.com

SkiWalking
5873 Lake Street
Glen Arbor, MI 49636
231-334-3080 or 877-SKIWALKING (754-9255)
www.skiwalking.com

Stride Poles
See Gabel

Swix Sport USA, Inc.
600 Research Drive
Wilmington, MA 01887
978-657-4820
www.swixsport.com
or
Swix Sport AS
Servicebox
N-2626 Lillehammer, Norway
(+47) 61 22 21 00
www.swixsport.no

Urban Poling Inc. (Canadian distributor for Exerstrider)
1015 Prospect Avenue
North Vancouver, BC
V7R 2M2, Canada
877-499-7999 or 604-980-1085
www.urbanpoling.com

OTHER EQUIPMENT & FURTHER RESOURCES

Adidas USA (footwear)
5055 North Greeley Avenue
Portland, OR 97217
800-448-1796
www.adidas.com

American Podiatric Medical Association, Inc.
9312 Old Georgetown Road
Bethesda, MD 20814-1621
301-581-9200
www.apma.org

Archives of Internal Medicine
American Medical Association
P.O. Box 10946
Chicago, IL 60654
800-262-2350 or 312-670-7827
http://archinte.ama-assn.org/

ASICS America Corporation (footwear)
29 Parker, Suite 100
Irvine, CA 92618
800-678-9435
www.asicsamerica.com

Brooks Sports Ltd (footwear)
The Courtyard, Nash Farm
Horsham Road, Steyning
West Sussex, UK BN44 3AA
(+44) 0 1903 817 009
www.brooksrunning.co.uk

CHEK Institute (holistic fitness trainer organization)
800-552-8789 or 760-477-2620
www.chekinstitute.com

Chung Shi USA (footwear)
http://chungshiusa.com
Chung Shi is imported into the USA exclusively for Foot Solutions and does not have an independent office in this country at this writing.
www.footsolutions.com

The Cooper Institute (health/wellness/medical)
12330 Preston Road
Dallas, TX 75230
972-341-3200
www.cooperinst.org

Earth Energetic (footwear)
135 Second Avenue
Waltham, MA 02451-1107
877-372-2814
www.earth.us

Easy Spirit (footwear)
c/o Jones Apparel Group Corporate Offices
180 Rittenhouse Circle
Bristol, PA 19007
215-785-4000
www.easyspirit.com (footwear), www.jny.com (corporate)

eVent Fabrics
c/o BHA Group, Inc.
8800 East 63rd Street
Kansas City, MO 64133
816-356-5515
www.eventfabrics.com

Fisher Center for Alzheimer's Research Foundation
One Intrepid Square
West 46th Street & 12th Avenue
New York, NY 10036
800-ALZINFO (259-4636)
www.alzinfo.org

**FootePath (instruction; specializing in overweight/
unfit beginners)**
6866 Lexington Drive
West Jordan, UT 84084
801-654-1059
www.footepath.org

Helsinki Polytechnic Stadia (sports academy)
PO Box 4000 Bulevardi 31
PL 4020
FI-00079 Metropolia, Finland
(+358) 20 783 5000
www.metropolia.fi/en/

The Heuga Center for Multiple Sclerosis
27 Main Street, Suite 303
Edwards, CO 81632
970-926-1290 or 800-367-3101
www.heuga.org

HD Medical (pulse oximeter)
5825 Edgemoor Drive
Houston, Texas, 77081
888-343-6334 or 713-344-0040
www.hdmedicaloutlet.com
Inov-8
See Revel Sports

INVISTA (CoolMax and other fabrics)
4123 East 37th Street North
Wichita, KS 67220
877-4-INVISTA (877-446-8478)
www.invista.com

Jacob Rohner AG (also see Sport Dinaco)
J. Schmidheinystrasse 23
CH - 9436 Balgach, Switzerland
(+41) 0 71 727 86 86
www.rohner-socks.com

Lands' End (Nordic Walking and other clothing)
1 Lands' End Lane
Dodgeville, WI 53595
800-800-5800
www.landsend.com

Lock Laces
Street Smart LLC
105 Sunset Drive
Glen Burnie, MD 21060
877-445-2237 or 410-590-7676
www.locklaces.com

Lowa Boots (footwear)
86 Viaduct Road
Stamford, CT 06907
888-335-LOWA
www.lowaboots.com

MBT/Masai Barefoot Technology (footwear)
Masai USA Corp.
515 North River Street, Unit D
Hailey, ID 83333
208-788-0883
or
Swiss Masai Marketing GmbH
St. Gallerstrasse 72
9325 Roggwil TG, Switzerland
www.swissmasaius.com

Mephisto France (footwear)
B.P. 50060
57401 Sarrebourg, France
(+33) 03 87 23 30 00
www.mephistousa.com
or
Mephisto USA
305 Seaboard Lane
Franklin, TN 37067
615-771-5900

Mizuno USA, Inc. (footwear)
4925 Avalon Ridge Parkway
Norcross, GA 30071
770-441-5553
www.mizunousa.com

New Balance Athletic Shoe, Inc.
Brighton Landing
20 Guest Street
Boston, MA 02135-2088
800-253-7463
www.newbalance.com

Nordic Walking Across America
See listing for T-Bone Productions

NordicPoleWalkingUSA, LLC
(instructional DVD and clothing)
P.O. Box 2162
Naples, FL 34102-2162
239-298-2612
www.nordicpolewalkingusa.com

Nordic Walking CO
177 Little Squaw Pass Road
Evergreen, CO 80439
303-674-2144
www.nordicwalkingco.com

The North Face, Inc. (footwear, clothing)
14450 Doolittle Drive
San Leandro, CA 94577
866-715-3223 (Warranty Department number)
www.thenorthface.com

Reebok International Ltd. (footwear)
1895 J.W. Foster Boulevard
Canton, MA 02021
781-401-5000
www.reebok.com

Reflectively Yours (reflective tape)
3 Ellen Lane
Glenville, NY 12302
518-399-9339
www.reflectivelyyours.com

Revel Sports (clothing, socks, accessories)
1903 Weston Avenue
Schofield, WI 54476
866-502-4125
www.revelsports.com

Rykä (women's footwear)
101 Enterprise, Ste. 100
Aliso Viejo, CA, 92653
888-834-rykä
www.ryka.com

Salomon Sports (footwear, patented releasable pole straps licensed to other manufacturers)
5055 North Greely Avenue
Portland, OR 97217
800-225-6850 or 971-234-7001
www.salomonsports.com
or
Salomon SA
Annecy Design Center
74996 Annecy Cedex 9
France
(+33) 0 4506 54141

Saucony, Inc. (footwear)
191 Spring Street
Lexington, MA 02420-9191
800-365-4933
www.saucony.com

SealSkinz Limited (waterproof socks)
36 Oldmedow Road
Hardwick Industrial Estate
King's Lynn
Norfolk PE30 4PP, United Kingdom
(+44) 0 1553 817990
www.sealskinz.com
or
c/o Danalco
1020 Hamilton Road
Duarte, CA 91010
800-868-2629
www.danalco.com

Shadow-Max Manufacturing, Inc. (dog leash harness)
440 Old Chesterfield Road
Winchester, NH 03470
603-239-6620
www.shadow-max.com

Spira (footwear)
110 Mesa Park Dr., Suite 200
El Paso, TX 79912
866-838-8640 or 915-838-8640
www.spirafootwear.com

The Sporn Company (dog leash harness)
274 West 86th Street
New York, NY 10024
800-223-1140
www.sporn.com

Sport Dinaco (Canadian importer of Rohner socks)
4330 Joseph Dubreuil
Lachine, QU H8T 3C4, Canada
514-636-8081
www.sportdinaco.com

SpringBoost USA Ltd. (footwear)
135 Beaver Street, Suite 305
Waltham, MA 02452
781-894 0009
www.springboost.com
or
SpringBoost S.A.
EPFL PSE A
1015 Lausanne
Switzerland
(+41) 21 694 01 80
www.springboost.com

STABILicers
(see 32North Corporation)

T-Bone Productions (promotions)
1207 River Ridge Drive
Asheville, NC 28803
828-298-4789
www.tbonerun.com

Teko (socks)
1435 Yarmouth St., Suite 102
Boulder, CO 80304
800-450-5784 or 303-449-7681
www.tekosocks.com

**32North Corporation
(STABILicers underfoot traction devices)**
6 Arctic Circle
Biddeford, ME 04007-5007
207-284-5010
www.32north.com

The Timberland Company (footwear)
200 Domain Drive
Stratham, NH 03885
603-772-9500
www.timberland.com

Tyless Shoelaces
P.O. Box 11205
Eugene, OR 97440
541-543-1080
www.tyless.com

YakTrax, LLC (underfoot traction devices)
9221 Globe Center Drive
Morrisville , NC 27560
800-446-7587
www.yaktrax.com

Books

Nordic Walking, by Malin Svensson. Published in 2009 by Human Kinestics (www.humankinestics.com).

Nordic Walking: A Total Body Experience, by Tim "T-Bone" Arem. Published in 2006.

Nordic Walking Equipment, Technique and Training, by Geert Hulshof. Published Wingstar B.V., 2005 in the Netherlands (English edition, 2006). Print on demand.

Nordic Walking Step by Step, by David Downer. Published by Nordic Walking Publications, 2006. Order from www.nordicwalkingstepbystep.com. It is available as a softcover book or as a downloadable e-book that can be printed out.

Original Nordic Walking, by Marko Kantaneva. Published in 2005 in hardcover by Pad-Centre and available as ane-book at www.poleabout.com or at www.nordicwalkingecommunity.com.

Stride and Glide: A Manual of Cross-Country Skiing and Nordic Walking, by Paddy Field and Stuart Montgomery. Published in 2006 in the U.K. by the publishers of Ski Nordic magazine as a print-on-demand book.

The Ultimate Nordic Walking Book, by Klaus Schwanbeck. Published in 2008 by Meyer & Meyer Sport (www.m-m-sports.com).

DVDs and Videos

In addition to instructional DVDs from various pole-makers, *Tele-Gym Nordic Walkin* is a 1 hour and 50 minute instructional DVD, in German, based on a Bavarian television series with Peter Schlickenrieder, a former Olympic cross-country skiing medalist and enthusiastic promoter of Nordic Walking in the German-speaking countries. The Tele-Gym Nordic Walking progression has been broken down into segments, and each part of the series can be viewed on-line at www.peter-schlickenrieder.de/245-Video.htm.